Exercise & Fitness

Jim Glenn

Medical Board

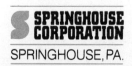

SPRINGHOUSE CORPORATION
SPRINGHOUSE, PA.

Program Director
Stanley Loeb

Clinical Director
Barbara McVan, RN

Art Director
John Hubbard

Editorial Services Supervisor
David Moreau

Production Manager
Wilbur Davidson

Editors
Jay Hyams
Susan Cass

The charter of the American Family Health Institute is to research and produce high-quality publications that enhance the health of individuals and their families. Essential to health are physical, emotional, and social well-being, not just the absence of illness or infirmity. The Institute's Medical Board has produced the *Health and Fitness* books to share up-to-date and authoritative information that can give readers greater personal control over their health maintenance.

Library of Congress Cataloging-in-Publication Data
Glenn, Jim.
  Exercise and fitness.
  (Health and fitness series)
  Includes index.
  1. Exercise.   2. Physical fitness.   3. Health.   I. Brunner, Lillian Sholtis.   II. American Family Health Institute. Medical Board. III. Title. IV. Series.   [DNLM: 1. Exertion—popular works.   2. Physical Fitness—popular works.   QT 255 G558e]
  RA781.G545   1986   613.7   85-30262
  ISBN 0-87434-024-1

The procedures and explanations given in this publication are based on research and consultation with medical and nursing authorities. To the best of our knowledge, these procedures and explanations reflect currently accepted medical practice; nevertheless, they can't be considered absolute and universal recommendations. For individual application, treatment suggestions must be considered in light of the individual's health, subject to a doctor's specific recommendations. The authors and the publisher disclaim responsibility for any adverse effects resulting directly or indirectly from the suggested procedures, from any undetected errors, or from the reader's misunderstanding of the text.

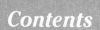

Contents

Exercise & Fitness

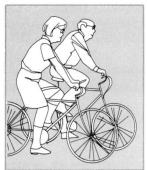

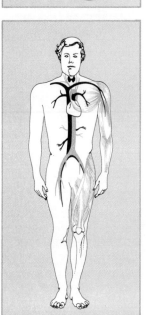

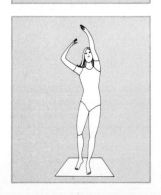

The fitness explosion

Who exercises and why?

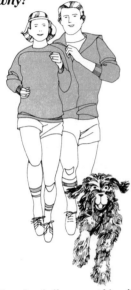

People of all ages and in all physical conditions exercise—a whole family may jog together. Why? To build stamina, lose weight, improve appearance, diminish stress, and reduce blood pressure, among others.

Fitness is a big industry. Statistics reflect two decades of surging sales—everything from running shoes to riding boots, sweatbands to sweat suits, and a host of other products associated with a fitter lifestyle. We know that people aren't just trying to fill up more leisure time; our national leisure has hovered around the same figure for some years. Americans are using sports facilities as never before, literally standing in line for their turns on the court. Magazines, books, films, and videotapes answer fitness questions and try perhaps to sell a few fitness fashions. Recently, celebrities vie as much for a place on the fitness bookshelf as for box office receipts. All the evidence says we're high-level fitness consumers.

- 70 million Americans exercise regularly.

- $35 billion are spent annually on physical activity.

- More than 300 marathons are run each year in the United States.

- Americans buy 19 million pairs of running shoes each year.

But who's becoming fit, and how fit are they? Surveys have suggested there are 35 million walking enthusiasts among us, 20 million cyclists, 10 million basketball players, 5 million weight lifters, 3 million martial artists, and maybe 25 million joggers. Such figures could be a little optimistic. Real information is hard to come by. Counting the number of jogging shoes sold and dividing by two doesn't necessarily equal the number of people who continue to jog regularly. We can be sure, however, that our variety of physical activities has reached a historic peak.

According to several surveys, fitness becomes a higher priority as income and education levels rise. Those in the 18 to 35 age group are more active than other groups. Men and women are equally likely to exercise, but in different ways. The real message in all this information, though, just might be that we're buying more equipment than we're using—or at least we aren't using it often enough. Data compiled by the President's Council on Fitness over the last quarter

How can you avoid injury?

To avoid injury:
* *Always warm up for a minimum of 10 to 20 minutes (see exercises on page 38).*
* *If you're tired, stop.*
* *If something hurts, stop.*
* *If you feel dizzy or nauseated, stop.*
* *Take your pulse at regular intervals.*
* *Cool down after exercising.*

A word about cautions

The cautions in this book are important, and you should heed them. But don't use the cautions as an excuse for not getting fit. Use this book to help you find an exercise program that's right for you.

century show we're as overweight now as we were 20 years ago. It has been argued that our downward-trending heart attack and stroke rate has a lot to do with lower-fat diets, medical advances, and less smoking. But no one is discounting exercise—even if many of us aren't exercising as regularly as we should, our exaggerated answers to fitness surveys show we've absorbed the right information.

What exercise can and can't do

As we'll see, almost any exercise is a good idea. And the reasons for regular exercise are overwhelmingly confirmed by research. Research also insists that even fit bodies have their limits. Not only is there a point of diminishing returns, but real danger may lie in a grueling excess of exercise effort.

While some claims made in behalf of exercise are still unclear, the large number of positive findings about regular exercise leaves no doubt: exercises *do* strengthen the heart, increase breathing efficiency, diminish stress, reduce blood pressure, burn away fat, improve appearance, and increase energy. Not the least of reported benefits is a heightened sexual vigor. Fitness is a bargain difficult to pass by.

The high cost of being unfit

We live within the limits of our bodies. If a physical activity is uncomfortable or painful to us, we'll avoid it. A sore back can take the pleasure from recreational activities and plague our working day, and yet chronic backache is often caused by nothing more complicated than lack of exercise for the spine's supporting muscles. A few simple exercises could make such a difference!

All too often, our inactive life-styles breed in us a fear of exertion. Such fears aren't entirely groundless —the executive age 40 who rushes headlong into an exercise program is apt to attempt too much too soon. Maybe he's punishing himself for neglecting his body during all those years of sitting behind a desk.

By middle age, many of us accomplish less, and attempt less, than we're really physically capable of. Anxiety, tension, and inertia mount. This isn't a healthful or hopeful state of affairs. No one can restore youthful energy, but exercise can rebuild confidence and vigor.

How to get started, how to stay with it

1. The decision to exercise
You may know you need more exercise, your doctor may have told you you need more exercise, or you may be interested in a certain sport or activity. Or perhaps you're just curious about the benefits of an exercise program.

2. Consult your doctor
If you decide to participate in any vigorous exercise program, you'll want to see your doctor first, particularly if you're over 30 or aren't accustomed to regular exercise.

3. Set up a program
Choose exercises you'll enjoy doing, establish a time of day, and find a convenient place. Perhaps you can find a partner—companionship makes many exercises more enjoyable.

4. Warm up and cool down
Include stretching exercises and proper warm-up and cool-down exercises in your program.

6. Strive for improvement
As you discover what you can do, you'll want to expand your goals. Your program will thus change to suit your abilities— and to serve you all your life.

5. Set goals
Some benefits of exercise aren't immediately apparent, and for those you'll need patience in the beginning. You'll be more likely to stay with your program if you set reasonable goals and work toward them.

Caution is in order

No matter how helpful you may find the encouragements, suggestions, and methods presented in this and other books, if you're over age 30 you shouldn't do any vigorous physical exercise without first consulting a doctor and having a physical examination. Indeed, no matter what your age, if you doubt your capacity for safe exercise, consult a doctor.

The more inactive your recent life-style, the more urgently you need to *ease* into exercise. An athletic past earns you no merit or special exemption if you're currently physically inactive.

Individuals convalescing or under treatment for illness must have medical advice and guidance. Heart patients, stroke victims, and diabetics should seek a doctor's opinion about any contemplated exercise program (if one has not already been recommended). High blood pressure, asthma, and obesity are additional conditions that require medical advice before you begin to exercise.

Finally, no sensible, health-minded person tries to "work off" an infection. The first aches and malaise aren't a signal to double your body's misery through the stress of exercise. Doing so may interfere with your body's immune response (ability to destroy invading microorganisms) to disease. Everything you can hope to achieve by exercising while sick is written in red ink as far as your health and fitness are concerned: don't do it.

2 Health, fitness, and exercise

Exercise and diet

If you're taking up an exercise program, try to eat a balanced diet of foods from the four food groups:
- *Dairy foods like milk and cheese*
- *Meats like beef, veal, and poultry*
- *Vegetables and fruits like green peppers and oranges*
- *Grains like breads, pasta, and rice*

Don't increase your intake of calories just because you're exercising—wait to see what happens to your weight.

Health, we agree, is the absence of illness. To a great degree we protect our health without the intervention of medicine: diet, hygiene, rest, and fitness can make major contributions to health. If this were all that health is made of, everyone would freely choose healthy life habits or unhealthy ones—or probably a personal mixture of both. And everyone would enjoy a sort of average health. Some choices aren't ours to make: heredity, infectious disease, environmental pollutants, and sheer accident can have large health consequences. Still, it's correct to believe that most people are in a position to make choices about health.

Can these always be informed choices? Does anyone *know* what's healthiest? The answer to both questions is a resounding *sometimes*. Medical ideas about diet seem to change with confusing frequency. We know for sure that modern medicine has revolutionized health, so why can't experts agree on the dietary benefit of something as simple as an egg? (Although an excellent protein source, egg yolks are relatively high in cholesterol.) If dietary science hasn't yet digested the egg, its findings have led us to lower salt and fat intake, away from certain preservatives, and to higher dietary fiber content. We're living longer as a result. Similarly, though the overall fitness message is clear, research still has a great many loose ends to tie up.

Fitness

Physical fitness isn't a single, ideal state of bodily affairs. Fitness to perform specific physical tasks—lifting a heavy weight, swimming the English Channel, or running a marathon—may require different kinds of body development. Underlying all physical activity, however, is a requirement for strength, flexibility, and endurance. Fitness, therefore, must have a great deal to do with muscles. Remember, the heart, too, is a muscle, easily the most important muscle in your body.

The degree to which any particular muscle is developed, whether some strength is to be traded for greater flexibility, and the intensity of exercise—these are components in any fitness program.

Body design

*The way your body is struc-
tured has a lot in common
with bridges, skyscrapers,
and airplanes. This means
your structure is the lightest possible for its high
strength. Like bridges, skyscrapers, and airplanes, you
can't twist and gyrate safely
under large loads. Therefore,
good exercises use twists
and rotations to develop
flexibility, not strength.
Strength exercises are safe
only when they utilize
balanced, linear motions.*

Exercise

Professional athletes are a generally fit group, and yet
emulating the athlete isn't necessarily a good idea.
Why? An athlete is not really paid to be fit but to perform. A major league pitcher designs his training
around one strong, flexible, overdeveloped arm.
(You'll find arguments about whether pitchers train
any more for endurance.) An oversized arm may well
not be your fitness aim, but neither is your fitness being measured in such specific performance terms as
earned run average and winning percentage. Most of
us desire a more general kind of fitness. Our performance is rated in body weight, pulse, blood pressure,
energy reserves, freedom from stress, improved
appearance—in other words, quality of life.

If an improved quality of life is your aim, your fitness
training will consist of a manageable exercise selec-
tion, regular workout sessions, perhaps some sports
participation, and an inclination to walk more, ride
less; to be more active, less sedentary.

Types of exercise

You can classify exercises. Body builders think of exercises by the muscle groups they wish to develop. Athletic coaches used to be satisfied with fairly simple
exercise categories: stamina, strength, flexibility.
These groupings are certainly useful, but they need
refinements.

You'll hear such terms as *aerobic* and *anaerobic*,
or maybe *isotonic, isokinetic,* and *isometric.* Each is a
way of describing exercise. In addition, exercise may
be *interval* training or *continuous.* Let's look at the
distinctions.

Aerobic and anaerobic exercise

Aerobic and anaerobic refer to the two basic ways in
which your muscles can produce energy. In aerobic
exercise, muscles "burn" fuels and oxygen, producing
little waste. Anaerobic burning consumes fuels without oxygen's presence; waste products quickly accu-
mulate in your muscles during anaerobic burning,
causing fatigue and sometimes pain.

Anaerobic activity takes place in the time before
enough oxygen can be carried to a working muscle—
the first 10 to 20 seconds of any exertion—or when the
need for strength is higher than simple oxygen burning can provide. Weight lifting is a high-strength,
short-duration exercise: it's mostly anaerobic. Any

Your exercise goals

*Are you interested in stam-
ina, strength, or flexibility?
If you're exercising for
fitness—to stay as young
and healthy as you can—
you'll need all three. Of
course, if you're 18 years
old, you might be more interested in building strength
than flexibility, and if you're
in your fifties, you might be
more interested in main-
taining your stamina and
flexibility. Whatever your
goals, you'll find enough information in this book to
plan your exercise program.*

Your heart and lungs

Unless you're exclusively interested in developing physical strength, for which anaerobic exercises are useful, you'll choose a program that concentrates on aerobic activities. These stimulate your heart and lungs. Aerobic exercises are important because not only might they make you look better, they'll also benefit your circulatory and respiratory systems.

start-and-stop activity calls for some degree of anaerobic energy. You've probably noticed that chores like shoveling snow or rearranging all the boxes stored in your garage are more fatiguing than steadier, lower-strength tasks such as vacuuming or pushing a power mower. This is because the more anaerobic chores require short bursts of strength. No sooner do your muscles gear up for smooth operation than the task is completed.

Aerobic exercise, in contrast, lasts at least long enough to bring the muscles into oxygen burning. And aerobic exercise doesn't tax your muscles to the straining point. Prime examples of aerobic activity are jogging, swimming, and walking. Pastimes such as dancing or even rope skipping qualify as good aerobic exercise so long as you continue them for 20 minutes or more at a time.

The whole point of aerobic exercise is to raise the efficiency of your muscles. That means making them stronger, getting more oxygen to them, and clearing away waste products more quickly. The muscle that benefits most is your heart: it becomes stronger as it works to pump blood to exercising muscles, and as your heart becomes stronger it circulates blood more easily, carrying more oxygen to all the muscles, including itself, and carrying away muscle waste products faster. Aerobic efficiency, therefore, is really cardiovascular efficiency (*cardiovascular* means the heart and circulatory system considered as a unit).

Aerobic training level

For best effects in aerobic exercise, you must work a little harder than what is comfortable for you, but a lot less than all-out exertion. The easiest way to find your aerobic training level is through taking your pulse during exercise. When your heart is beating at between 70 and 85 percent of its maximum rate, you'll achieve very good conditioning.

As you can see from the chart (on page 11), your heart's maximum rate (in beats per minute) depends upon your age. The maximum rate falls slowly and steadily as you grow older. Please note that this maximum is nothing more than a measure, on average, of what a healthy heart muscle can do. It's neither an "unsafe" nor a "safe" level of exertion—your safety in exercise depends upon a medical checkup and your doctor's advice.

How to find your aerobic training level

To find your aerobic training level, you'll need to take your pulse. Find the pulse point in your wrist; explore for it with your fingertips. A pulse can also be felt in your neck. Usually the wrist pulse is strongest, but if you take the carotid (neck) pulse, be sure to feel for it low on your neck. You can interrupt blood supply to the brain by applying pressure higher up on the carotid.

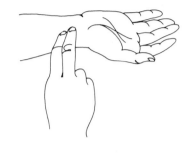

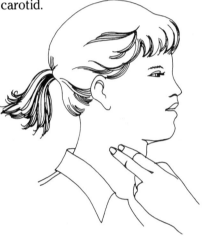

Age	70 percent	85 percent
20	23	28
25	23	28
30	22	27
35	22	26
40	21	26
45	20	25
50	20	24
55	19	23
60	19	23
65	18	22
70	18	21

Having found your pulse, use your watch to count the number of pulse beats in a 10-second interval. Then refer to the chart. Find your age in the left column. Read across to find your 70 percent and 85 percent of maximum pulse rates during a 10-second reading.

For the most beneficial results, maintain your pulse during exercise between the 70 and 85 percent figures.

If you want to know what your 1-minute pulse rate should be, multiply your 10-second count by 6.

Don't exercise at your maximum heart rate but in the 70 to 85 percent range—the "zone" indicated in the chart. You won't achieve any more fitness benefit by exercising at your body's upper limits than by exercising within the aerobic zone. In fact, only competitive athletes, such as professional marathon runners, train constantly at punishing levels of intensity—and they must guard against the unhealthy effects of overtraining (for example, chronic fatigue, joint and bone problems).

Exercise at less than maximum levels is called submaximal. Research shows aerobic improvements begin with exercise at as low as 60 percent of maximum heart rate, but little more is achieved above 85 percent. Exercise anywhere within this range has good fitness value. However, the quickest fitness gains appear to occur between 70 and 85 percent. And, as you might expect, submaximal exercise at 70 percent of your capacity requires somewhat longer workouts to match the results of shorter sessions at 85 percent capacity.

Aerobic and anaerobic exercise

Aerobic exercise is an uninterrupted exercise of a muscle or group of muscles that burns oxygen in the muscle tissues. Because the exercise is continuous and fairly regular, it doesn't tax muscles to exhaustion, as you know—think about how long you can walk or, if you're in condition, jog or swim. In contrast, an anaerobic exercise—for example, weight lifting— works a muscle or muscle group briefly and intensely to the point of exhaustion. Anaerobic exercises are too brief to burn significant oxygen in muscle tissues. Because they're performed longer than anaerobic exercises, aerobic increase the efficiency and strength of your heart.

Anaerobic and aerobic activity compared

Exercising to raise your anaerobic capability—for bursts of heavy work, peak strength—also raises your aerobic capacity, but not very much. And you won't get very far with anaerobic training if you're not already aerobically conditioned.

Aerobic and anaerobic exercises bring different kinds of benefits. Competitive shorter-distance swimmers, for example, need high anaerobic power; long-distance swimmers, too, need the extra performance, that last ounce, of an anaerobic boost. Still, in all swimmers' training schedules, aerobics takes priority. That's because a strong heart and good circulation are the very basis of fitness, for those who compete and for those who don't.

Isokinetic and isotonic exercise

Both these terms refer to what muscles do when they move against a resistance; both are dynamic effort. Isokinetic exercise is a little specialized: it usually requires equipment (with springs and levers and such) that keeps muscles under the same high tension across the entire range of a particular motion. When an isokinetic machine, such as a Nautilus, isn't available, isokinetic exercise requires a partner, someone to match you resistance for resistance—as in an arm-wrestling bout.

Isotonic exercise is everything else: running, walking, swimming, calisthenics, dancing, cross-country skiing, and nearly anything you do when you move. Isotonic exercise is rhythmic, aerobic, and develops muscular endurance.

Movable objects, immovable objects

Isometric exercises involve muscles working against an immovable object. Pushing against a wall is an example of an isometric exercise. Following the one-time exertion of the muscle, no further movement is possible. Working out on a Nautilus machine is a form of isokinetic exercise: muscles are working against resistance. Exertion continues against the muscle throughout the entire range of motion.

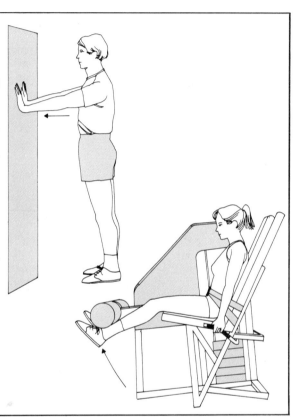

Isometric exercise

Muscle work against an unmoving object is isometric, also called static effort. Isometrics were highly thought of in the 1960s, but they do little to improve the heart and circulation since these exercises are principally anaerobic. Although isometrics increase the strength and size (but not the endurance) of muscles, some researchers believe that spiking blood pressure, which occurs during isometric exertion, is a negative feature. For this reason, isometrics aren't generally recommended for older people, and certainly not for those with high blood pressure.

Switching your body's power sources

Sprinting is an interesting example of the way anaerobic and aerobic processes work. In competition, sprinters nearly always slow down before they reach the finish line. They start the race burning anaerobic fuel, which gives them maximum speed. But their anaerobic waste products are building, even as their muscles are making the changeover to a more constant, aerobic energy supply. Aerobic energies aren't enough to sustain the highest speeds, so the pace slackens noticeably after about 10 seconds. You might say, the finish line lies in the transition zone between anaerobic and aerobic metabolism.

Why boredom?

What if you're bored by 20 minutes of continuous running? You can spend your exercise time of 20 to 30 minutes in more than one way. If you enjoy doing the exercise at a constant pace for the full period of time, that's fine. But you can also use a slower pace for 5 to 10 minutes and alternate with a faster pace for 5 to 10 minutes. Some people find the alternating less effortful and more interesting. Take your choice.

Squeezing a tennis ball for a few seconds is isometric; so is holding a weight out in front of you or pulling on a stuck window. Waterskiing and downhill skiing are both highly isometric sports; gymnastics, weight lifting, and horseback riding have isometric components.

Interval versus continuous training

You may choose to work out strenuously for 30 minutes at a time or more. Or you may prefer shorter, intense efforts interrupted with slack, recovery intervals. Experts sometimes split hairs when advancing the merits of one method over the other. Many people freely combine continuous and interval training in whatever mix they find most agreeable. (Experts also disagree about the best ratio of effort to rest for interval training—anywhere from 30 seconds to 5 minutes of intense work, followed by at least an equivalent coasting period.)

Experts do agree about these points:

Interval training
• Appropriate interval training may achieve beneficial cardiovascular results a little faster than continuous training.

• Interval training is less strenuous than continuous exertion. Therefore older and more sedentary people should consider it.

• Many people find 30 to 40 minutes of jogging or swimming—or an hour's walk—quite boring. Interval training offers variety.

Continuous training
• Continuous training develops muscle endurance. Long-distance runners *must* run long distances in practice to be at all competitive.

American runners were for decades poor finishers in the marathon. That's because they used chiefly interval training in their conditioning. Following the example of Jim Ryun, they were soon logging 100 miles and more each week in practice. And they began to win marathons.

• Many people relax with the rhythm of a long, steady workout. Peace and inner quiet are, needless to say, a healthful bonus. Of course, you may find tranquility elsewhere, in other forms of exercise or recreation.

• Continuous training, particularly distance running,

Exercise and calories

If you count the number of calories burned during your 20 to 30 minute exercise session, you might find the results depressing. Cheer up: regular exercise pays off because your body continues to burn extra calories for hours after you've ended your exercise. This surprising benefit may make counting burned calories a bit more complicated, but it means you'll lose more weight than simple math suggests.

Will exercising reduce your hunger?

Many experts say that you'll be less hungry after you exercise, but some regular exercisers don't find that to be true. If you're hungry after you exercise, don't sit down to eat immediately. Let your body cool down thoroughly. In the meantime, you can control a strong craving for food by drinking vegetable and fruit juices.

carries with it a higher risk of eventual injury, usually to an overworked joint or tendon—unless you vary your exercises.

Having now classified exercises by power source (aerobic, anaerobic), by muscle action (isotonic, isokinetic, isometric), by intensity (submaximal), and by training method (interval, continuous), let's compare some exercises.

Comparing exercises

How can we say, for example, that dancing a Virginia reel equals 5 minutes of bicycling at 9 miles an hour—and that's a scientific fact? Obviously, only numbers can be exactly equal to one another. We need some kind of meaningful numbers to describe exercise effort if we wish to compare unlike physical activities.

All physical effort requires fuel and oxygen to power your muscles. The greater the muscular effort, the larger the amounts of fuel and oxygen you use. Thus, we can compare different kinds of exercise by measuring either fuel or oxygen consumption during various exercises. If we're measuring oxygen, the number we want is expressed as the volume of oxygen (in milliliters) consumed each minute per kilogram (2.2 pounds) of body weight. A figure given in ml O_2/kg.min is, therefore, the *cost* of any exercise. This cost serves equally well to describe the physical effort of running a race, shopping for groceries, singing a difficult aria, or anything else you use your muscles to do.

In addition to looking at the oxygen burned, we also can compute what the oxygen is burning—the fuels your body derives from foods. In this case we want to know how many calories of heat oxygen and its consumed fuels create. An activity's calorie cost is perhaps the most familiar measure of exercise effort. Calories burned, as we all know, mean weight lost. There are 3,500 calories in a pound of fat; that translates into a 40-mile walk, an 8-hour tennis match, or maybe a solid 50 hours of watching TV. As you can see, one pound of fat represents a lot of energy. You can't work it off all at once.

The mere *cost* of exercise should not be confused with its *value*. Value is a broader concept—not easily expressed in numbers. Weight lifters and ballet dancers may exercise at the same energy cost, but they find little value in using each other's exercise routines interchangeably. Furthermore, identical exercise costs may produce in various individuals very different levels of satisfaction, of body conditioning, even of pain. These, too, are things that count in the value of exercise.

Energy costs of various activities

Activities listed here are measured in thousands of calories—*kilocalories*, or just Kcal—burned each hour. One calorie is such a small amount of heat energy that no one uses anything smaller than the kilocalorie when speaking of body output. Always assume that *calorie*, when it relates to food or the body, means large calorie.

All of the values here are for a person weighing about 150 pounds; add 10 calories an hour for every 5 pounds of your weight above 150 pounds. Subtract 10 calories for every 5 pounds of your weight under 150.

Activity	Energy cost (calories an hour)	Activity	Energy cost (calories an hour)
sleeping	70	cycling (6 mph)	320
watching TV	75	volleyball	320
standing	85	walking (4 mph)	320
knitting	85	square dancing	340
talking	100	soft-shoe dance	360
driving a car	120	horseback riding	360
polishing shoes	130	swimming	360–700
playing cards	140	badminton	380
walking (2 mph)	180	ice skating	400
bowling	210	tennis	420
playing pool	220	waterskiing	440
golfing	220	shoveling snow	460
waltzing	240	squash	520
calisthenics	280	skiing (downhill)	600
baseball	280	cycling (12 mph)	620
table tennis	280	jogging (5.5 mph)	650
mopping	300	skiing (cross-country)	840
weeding	320	marathon	920

(These figures are necessarily approximations; everyone performs a little differently.)

Clumsy isn't necessarily bad

Figures giving the energy cost of physical effort are always approximations. That's because everyone performs a little differently at, say, tennis, or waltzing, or polishing shoes. Some people exert themselves more than others, and some are less efficient, which means they'll use more energy in what they do.

Please note that just burning up calories doesn't insure fitness. Professional chess players, a notoriously short-lived bunch, burn calories at the rate of 300 calories an hour—equivalent to light gymnastics. Indeed, grand masters may push themselves to physical exhaustion. These calories, however, aren't spent in physical conditioning but consumed in brain metabolism. This may keep their minds in good shape; their bodies certainly don't benefit.

3 Your body and exercise

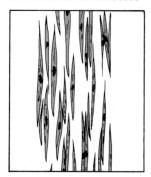

Smooth

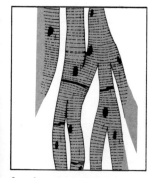

Involuntary striated

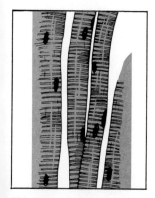

Voluntary striated

Your body has three kinds of muscle: smooth muscle (stomach, intestines), involuntary striated muscle (heart), and voluntary striated muscle (skeletal muscles). In exercise we're concerned with striated muscles, both the ones we consciously control and the heart, for whose benefit we exert ourselves.

Fuel
Muscles derive working energy from splitting a chemical bond in something called ATP (adenosine triphosphate), forming ADP (adenosine diphosphate) and a leftover phosphate. Energy is released when the bond breaks. Then, using fuels (sugars, fats, a very little protein) and oxygen, ADP is recombined with its leftover phosphate to start the cycle over again—it's called the Krebs cycle. This somewhat simplified account describes what goes on in a muscle.

Neither is oxygen absolutely necessary to start muscle work. As you know, though, oxygen arrives to an exercising muscle within 10 to 20 seconds. Until that point, anaerobic energy depends upon glycogen (a sugar) and ATP, which produces energy but leaves lactic acid as a waste product. Fatigue and pain increase as lactic acid builds up in a muscle. The waste products are cleared away by the bloodstream.

Muscles endure much longer when they are fueled aerobically, with oxygen. The same sugars and fats and ATP *with* the addition of enough oxygen produce only water and carbon dioxide wastes, which don't interfere with muscle work.

Muscle fiber
The basic unit of muscle activity is the muscle fiber. It's a single, narrow cell running uninterrupted along the whole muscle length. Fibers are paralleled by nerves (which receive activation signals) and capillaries. Most of the moving parts of muscles are made of two rodlike proteins, myosin and actin.

Filaments of myosin and actin are gathered into large bundles called myofibrils, which in turn are gathered into one muscle fiber. Though myosin and actin

A muscle and its fibers

The smallest working unit of a muscle is the myofibril. Within each myofibril, contraction takes place when two rodlike proteins, myosin and actin, pull past each other with a sliding motion. Thousands of myofibrils (10,000 to the inch) are strung together lengthwise to make a sarcomere. Sarcomeres, in turn, are gathered together to form one complete muscle fiber. Each fiber, with its own blood and nerve supply, is really a single body cell, though a very long one.

Parallel muscle fibers are packed together in one muscle bundle, and the bundles themselves are grouped together into a final array—which is a complete muscle, such as a biceps, calf, or pectoral muscle. Encasing muscle bundles and attaching them to bone is a versatile connective tissue. This tissue grows extremely tough at the junction of bone and muscle—where it's called a tendon—but becomes more resilient along a muscle's length.

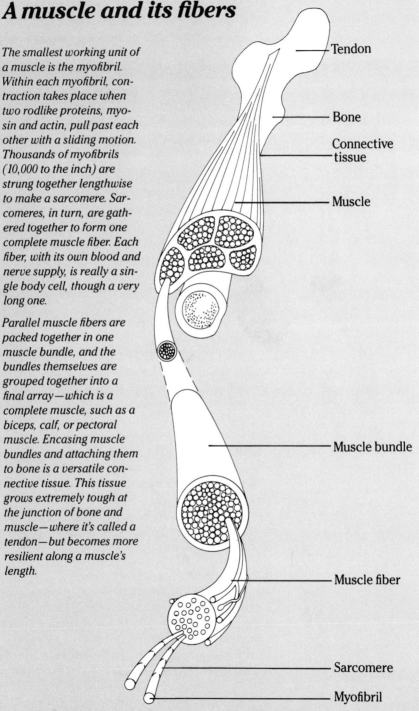

Tendon

Bone

Connective tissue

Muscle

Muscle bundle

Muscle fiber

Sarcomere

Myofibril

A high-protein diet myth

High-protein diets aren't needed to fuel muscles. Muscle cells depend primarily on carbohydrates for fuel, not proteins. The best carbohydrates for fuel are found in fruits, unrefined grains, pasta, and breads. These are digested more slowly than sugars and provide a steady source of fuel for muscles.

never touch each other, energy released in ATP splitting gives them an electrical attraction; they move to overlap each other in a parallel, sliding action. (Each parallel array of myosin and actin is only a few micrometers long; thousands of such units, or sarcomeres, form a muscle chain running the whole fiber length.)

Note that the proteins don't actually contract or "curl up"—they slide by each other when activated and back again when relaxed (with the help of two other proteins). The net effect to muscle fiber, as its thousands of sarcomere segments shorten themselves, is a powerful contraction. The force is multiplied by gathering thousands of fibers into muscle bundles, and a few bundles into each complete muscle.

The sheathing around a muscle turns subtly into tendon at each end, to attach it to bone. All muscles terminating in the same tendons make up one muscle group.

Thus, when you bring a large muscle, such as the calf muscle, into action, thousands of fibers (and millions of sarcomere segments) are shortening themselves in unison.

Muscle fibers are of two types, distributed in various proportions in different muscles (and in different people). Fast-twitch fibers are thick with few capillaries. They're also quick and strong but fatigue easily. Slow-twitch fibers contract more slowly but have much more endurance than fast-twitch fibers. Slow-twitch fibers, with a richer blood supply, seem better equipped to work aerobically.

The number of fibers in a particular muscle, and the distribution of fast- and slow-twitch fibers, is genetically determined. No amount of exercise will grow extra fibers or transform one kind into another. Exercise will improve muscular efficiency and strength. However, muscles will grow with exercise as individual fibers increase in diameter. (This effect is less marked in women because certain hormones limit muscle growth.)

One of a kind

The heart, about the size of an adult man's fist, pumps without interruption from before you're born until you die. While your heart's health isn't entirely determined by you, you can do good things for it by exercising reasonably and regularly. The more efficient the heart's performance, the easier its job, and exercise will improve its efficiency.

The heart

The heart's muscle type is maximized for endurance. In addition to pumping oxygenated blood to the rest of the body and used blood to the lungs, the heart must also maintain its own fresh blood supply.

The nervous system controls all these activities automatically. Briefly, these processes are classified as

(continued on page 22)

Major muscle groups

As you look at the body's major muscles, remember that muscles work only as they contract: muscles never push, they pull.

Muscles that move your limbs are either flexors or extensors. A flexor, attached to the inside of a joint, moves a limb inward, toward the trunk. Extensors do the opposite. The most familiar pair are probably biceps and triceps. The biceps, a flexor, pulls your forearm toward your shoulder.

Frontview

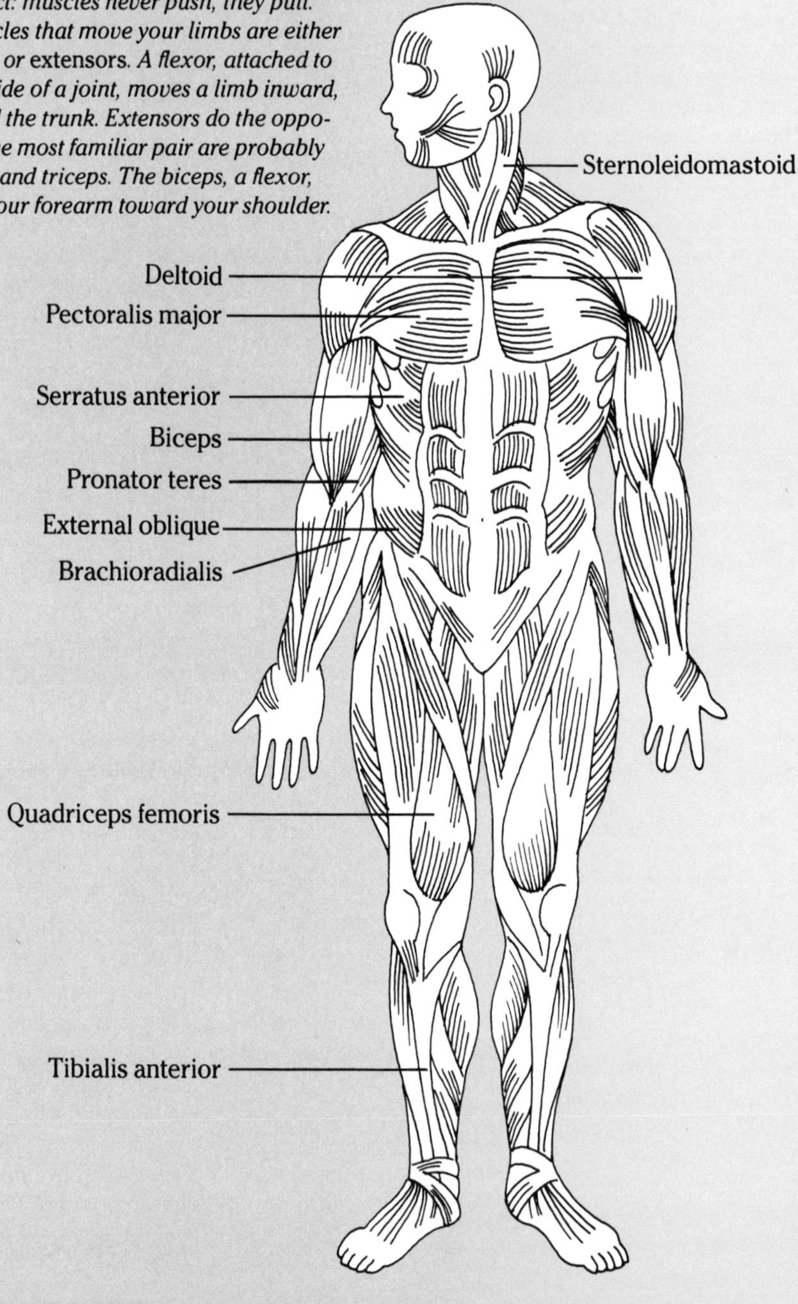

Sternoleidomastoid

Deltoid

Pectoralis major

Serratus anterior

Biceps

Pronator teres

External oblique

Brachioradialis

Quadriceps femoris

Tibialis anterior

Attached to a lever point behind the elbow, the triceps, an extensor, pulls the forearm down and away from the shoulder.

If you understand where your muscles are and what they do, you can devise exercises for specific muscles. Use the principles of overload and repetition, combined with the contracting motion peculiar to an individual muscle. But avoid anything that feels like overextending or that causes pain.

Backview

Trapezius

Triceps

Latissimus dorsi

Brachioradialis

Gluteus maximus

Semitendinosus

Semimembranosus

Biceps femoris

Gastrocnemius

Achilles' tendon

Your heart

Your heart is really two pumps in one muscular bundle. Each pump consists of two pumping chambers: the artrium and the ventricle. Blood entering the heart's right side has already been circulated through your body and is low in oxygen. This blood enters the right atrium from your body's two largest veins, the inferior and and superior vena cava. The right ventricle pumps blood through the pulmonary arteries to your lungs to pick up oxygen.

Oxygenated blood travels from the lungs to the left atrium by way of the pulmonary veins. In the final step, the left ventricle pumps oxygenated blood through the aorta to the rest of your body.

The heart, too, needs a supply of oxygen-rich blood; it's provided through the coronary arteries, which encircle the heart, ensuring the richest possible blood supply to this most vital organ.

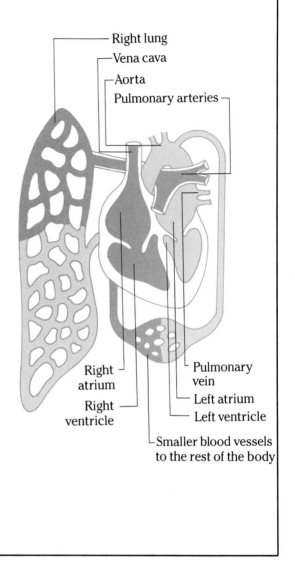

Right lung
Vena cava
Aorta
Pulmonary arteries
Right atrium
Right ventricle
Pulmonary vein
Left atrium
Left ventricle
Smaller blood vessels to the rest of the body

either sympathetic or parasympathetic. The sympathetic system stimulates, the parasympathetic slows. When we speak of a "surge of adrenaline," we refer to one sympathetic effect. Our sympathetic responses seem to originate as a primitive survival strategy. These responses prepare us for "fight or flight."

Too much sympathetic activity tends to wear out parts of the circulatory system and the heart itself. Such things as anxiety and tension increase sympathetic response, hence the well-documented relationship between stress and heart disease. Most exercise

What do the numbers mean?

What does it mean when someone says his blood pressure is 120 over 75? The top number records the pressure caused in your arteries as blood surges through each time your heart pumps. The bottom number records the fall of pressure as your heart rests between beats.

has the effect of enhancing parasympathetic activity and actually lowering mental stress.

If the heart is made to feel a little oxygen-starved, new capillaries form around the heart to increase flow (collateral circulation). During vigorous exercise the heart senses an oxygen shortage (hypoxia) and initiates new capillary formation. Collateral circulation increase takes months to develop, hence exercise must be somewhat vigorous and regular to achieve this result. In theory, the availability of collateral circulation gives protection to your heart during sudden artery blockage. No evidence suggests this theory is wrong—very much to the contrary—but opinions differ about its proportionate contribution to lower heart attack rates among exercisers.

The circulatory system

The body's blood vessels should circulate blood with a minimum of friction and obstruction. If vessels narrow, constricting blood flow, blood pressure must go up just to get enough blood through them. Of course, blood pressure can go only so high—either the heart will pump no harder or a vessel wall will give way at some weak point (aneurysm). Either of these occurrences is catastrophic.

What is blood pressure? How is it controlled? During the heart's pumping action blood is forced at highest pressure away from the heart and through branching arteries. This pressure is called systolic. Between heartbeats, pressure falls to a minimum. This pressure is called diastolic. We usually express blood pressure giving both numbers, systolic first, then the diastolic—for example, 110/70 or 130/80. Roughly speaking, the diastolic pressure gives an indication of the circulatory system's resistance to flow. The higher the diastolic number, the higher systolic pressure has to be to keep blood moving. Your blood pressure may go up and down many times a day as your moods and activities change.

What happens at high altitude

Thinner air at high altitudes means less oxygen in each breath you take. The body can adjust to lowered oxygen, but it takes time. These adjustments can never quite match those of someone actually born and raised at a particular altitude. (Subtle changes take place even before birth for high-altitude natives.)

Special considerations
When you exercise, you should take into account factors other than how you feel or how much time you have, including:

• *The weather. If it's extremely hot and humid, exercise will be more effortful, and you'll need to be aware of heat exhaustion and heat stroke signs. If it's very cold, you'll need to dress in layers and be aware of frostbite signs.*

• *The altitude. If you're at a high elevation, you'll be able to accomplish less because your heart will have to work harder to keep your blood circulating. You'll need to watch for signs of mountain sickness.*

Your body's chief response to altitude is to shrink the blood's fluid content. Thus more oxygen-carrying red blood cells are packed into the same blood volume—about 15 percent more at 7,000 feet. Your heart will have to work at slightly higher output, keeping the smaller blood volume circulating faster. Doing too much too quickly may cause "mountain sickness": faintness, weakness, headache, perhaps euphoria, and rapid, gasping breaths.

Initial adaptation takes from 2 to 3 weeks. Physically conditioned and unconditioned individuals adapt at the same rate. Not for months does the body begin producing higher numbers of red blood cells. And lung enlargement takes years, if it happens at all. Acclimation is never really finished.

In a sense, at higher altitudes your heart is performing constant aerobic exercise. Athletes have tried to take advantage of this, training at higher elevations to improve performance at sea level. Results are unclear; if an advantage exists, it is nearly undetectable.

The brain

Exercise won't enlarge your brain or make you smarter. But it'll keep oxygen flowing to your brain at a reasonably low blood pressure. Insofar as exercise improves heart efficiency, the brain benefits. Insofar as exercise reduces stress, builds confidence, and performance, your psyche benefits.

More about the nervous system: tranquilizers?

The brain can respond to extremes of exertion by releasing pain killers. These substances, norepinephrine and beta-endorphin, may produce euphoria, a "high." For some people, this adds an inducement to exercise. They find exertion euphoric and addictive. Nearly everyone agrees, however, that exercise, with or without euphoria, has real benefits—so long as fitness "addicts" don't push themselves into overexertion and injury.

Exercise also has a measurable tranquilizing effect on the body. One study found that administering 400 milligrams of meprobamate, a minor tranquilizer, duplicates the relaxation (in muscle tension) of a vigorous workout. Such results are not as exact as they seem: tension arises from many causes, and people don't respond equally to exercise or to meprobamate, for that matter. However, since exercise doesn't have unwanted side effects, like some tranquilizers, it's an attractive alternative.

Highly competitive activity and constant high-intensity exertion are sometimes associated with an *increase* in stress. No one can say for sure whether higher stress lies in the nature of competition or of competitors. Or which mixture of both is apt to be most stressful.

Women and exercise

Basic fitness is an important goal for men and women. Exercise benefits are very similar for both—particularly in aerobic capacity—but biochemical and physical differences suggest a different emphasis in conditioning activities.

Hormones

The female hormone estrogen limits muscle growth. Estrogen may also be responsible for generally lower fat levels in the blood. Women tend also to have a more desirable blood ratio of high-density (HDL) to low-density (LDL) fat carriers (lipoproteins). These are probable factors in the significantly lower heart disease rate among women. (Evidence for this "protection" disappears after menopause.)

Menarche and menstrual cycle

Some girls engaged in vigorous physical training (such as track, ballet, swimming) experience a delayed menstrual onset (menarche). The long-term effects of a later menarche are unknown. (Even without exercise, girls who live at higher altitudes reach menarche later.) Yet intense training *is* associated with disturbances of the menstrual cycle. Girls who begin training before menarche, particularly competitive runners, experience the greatest problems. Those who enter energetic endurance activities after menarche experience the least menstrual disturbance.

Menstrual function usually returns to normal shortly after the individual ceases or even reduces intense exercising. But intense exercise is only one of many reasons for menstrual abnormalities: youth, stress, weight loss, illness, and personal history are important factors.

Researchers also find a strong relationship between body fat percentage and menstrual function. When a woman's body fat drops below a certain percentage of her total weight, hormone levels are affected. Rapid

Watch your iron!
Exercise doesn't seem to increase vitamin requirements; however, women may be in short supply of the mineral iron, especially if they are active. Iron deficiency can impair athletic performance and lead to anemia and fatigue. Be sure you're getting enough iron in the foods you eat. Foods high in iron include beef liver, lima beans, apricots, broccoli, spinach, peas, raisins, and chicken.

Getting and keeping your minerals

Though your body is very good at maintaining the proper mineral balance for your needs, strenuous exercise may deplete your mineral stores somewhat faster than normal. Of course, exercise also helps your body make best use of tissue-building and energy-releasing minerals. So eat well, exercise well, and don't exhaust yourself.

weight loss exaggerates the effect. For these and other reasons, women should avoid crash diets and lighten their training programs when activity is causing too steep a weight loss.

Exercise and pregnancy

Women who exercise regularly and enjoy this activity may certainly continue during the first and second trimesters of pregnancy. They will, of course, want regular checkups and medical opinion. Be advised, however, that pregnancy is *not* a good time to begin an exercise program.

When intense exercise is suspected as the cause of menstrual disturbance, women are usually advised not to attempt pregnancy until exercise levels are reduced and regular menstrual function returns.

Getting rid of fat

Fat is, among other things, a form of stored body energy. Unfortunately, we store this energy in highly visible ways around the waist, thighs, upper arms, and elsewhere. The obvious solution is to convert fat back into energy via exercise. But fat serves also as insulation and protection to parts of the body. This is particularly true in women.

The body-wide fat distribution is highly individual. We inherit a certain body shape. Women generally have a higher ratio of fat to muscle than men. Reducing your fat levels much below those where your body works best is not a good idea. Not only will your hormonal balance be disturbed—with a host of physiological consequences—but some people can actually lose essential nonfat tissue.

The body's biochemistry may choose, at certain critical fat levels, to sacrifice other body materials—such as tendons—instead of fat. In other words, fat reserves are protected or grudgingly used if they fall too quickly or too far. As you exercise and watch others, you'll see that for each body type there is a reasonable range of development and improved appearance.

Demineralization

Women are at higher risk than men of losing bone minerals and suffering from a condition called osteoporosis. Research suggests that exercise helps build your bones as well as your muscles. But you can overdo, too. Long, punishing endurance exercises, particularly intense jogging, can speed up demineralization in women.

The wise exerciser takes a preventive step by recognizing that he or she needs a good daily supply of calcium from milk or cheese, yogurt, or green leafy vegetables.

Weight lifting for women

Women and men benefit from repetition exercises with lower weights. Such exercise enhances strength and endurance while giving definition to the body, improving appearance. Lifting heavier weights, as a competitive sport or a pastime, is a personal choice. Peak strength increases with heavier lifting, but so does risk of injury. No one should undertake rigorous or heavy lifting without a knowledgeable instructor's guidance.

A word about body types

Systematic study of body shapes has been with us for centuries. Some of this research has pointed to valuable further inquiry, and some is pure quackery. Generally, body shapes come in three types, marked by relative fatness, muscularity, and slightness of build. The point of classifying shapes is to make predictions about physical qualities.

Two unfortunate tendencies seem to accompany an enthusiasm for body-typing: (1) assumptions that an "ideal" or best body type exists and (2) belief that body type determines personality, intelligence, or character traits.

The best of body-typing measurements were performed by William Sheldon. His theory of *somatotypes* is the most familiar to us. Individuals are described by a three-digit number, rating body shape and structure on three scales (each ranging from 1 to 7): *endomorph* (rounded, fat), *mesomorph* (square, muscular), and *ectomorph* (slightly built, slender). A pure mesomorph, for example, would rate 171, or lowest on the endomorph and ectomorph scales and highest on the mesomorph. Almost no one, however, rates as a single, pure somatotype.

Sheldon's method is useful in assessing various physical capacities. After all, physique *is* genetic evidence of some kind. Mesomorphs *are* stronger than ectomorphs; endomorphs *aren't* good at long-distance running. Even longevity, which is partially genetically determined, may be vaguely related to body types. But somatotypes can't be pushed very far in describing mental traits, as Sheldon himself concluded.

Concentrate on what you can do

Don't be obsessed with your body type. Remember that if you're slight and slender or rounded and full or squarish and muscular, you can't change these fundamentals. But in no case are you guaranteed to be attractive or unattractive. What almost everyone will admire is the energy and attitude you'll convey to others if you're in good physical condition.

Body types

You probably won't recognize yourself here. That's because these illustrations show the extremes of each somatotype. Most people have mixed features of each type.

Ectomorph **Endomorph** **Mesomorph**

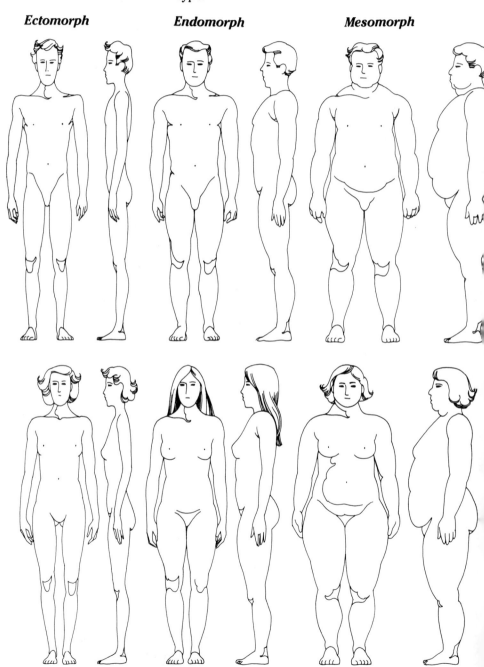

Getting ready

No doubt you already have some idea about your physical condition. Everyday exertions—climbing stairs, moving furniture, gardening—signal to you your body's general fitness. To make meaningful measurements of yourself, however, you will want to use a standard test.

Exercise physiologists and doctors would test you on a treadmill. Walking speeds and uphill grades can be precisely controlled. During and after a test, moreover, various machines can take note of your blood pressure, heart action, oxygen uptake, breathing volume, and so on. Tests of this sort are called stress tests —they measure your body's cardiovascular response to exertion.

The results are far from definitive. They're not reliable enough to make any certain diagnosis, positive or negative, about the presence of heart disease; doctors use them as part of a larger diagnostic scheme. But stress tests do measure your exercise capacity. The test you'll use here resembles a stress test: you'll em-

Stress tests

Your body responds to exercise by increasing its demand for oxygen— the result of increased breathing, heart output, and use of oxygen by your tissues. Stress tests measure these changes by monitoring heart rate, blood pressure, use of oxygen, and other body functions. Thus, if you take a stress test, you may find yourself connected to various devices such as an EKG (electrocardiogram), which produces a graphic record of the electrical current generated by the heartbeat.

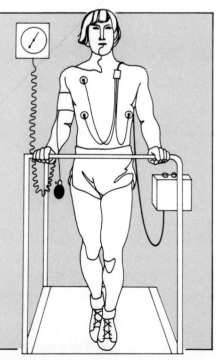

ploy a standard piece of equipment (an 8-inch step), a standard measure (your pulse rate), and a very small amount of exertion.

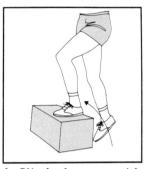

1. Climb the step with your left foot.

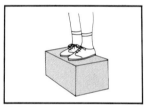

2. Bring your right foot up.

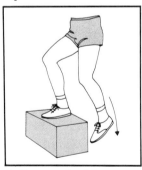

3. Descend with your left foot.

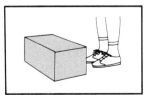

4. Bring your right foot down.

The self test

Find a step, low bench, or very sturdy stool 7 or 8 inches high. Measure your pulse before starting. If it's over 100, you shouldn't attempt this exercise. Climb the step with your left foot; bring your right foot up. Descend with your left foot and then your right. Continue this one-step climb and descent for 1 minute. Keep a step count by the number of times you bring your left foot up. Thus, each up-and-down repetition counts as 1.

Try to complete 24 steps in 1 minute. Then sit down and take your pulse 1 full minute after you complete the test. Check your pulse on this chart:

	Men	**Women**
Excellent	under 68	under 76
Good	68-79	76-85
About average	80-89	86-94
Below average	90-99	95-109
Poor	over 100	over 100

If your pulse is higher than the average upper limit shown in this chart, you're probably less physically fit than the average person in your age group. You'll benefit most from beginning a regular fitness program. Results in the average range, too, should be improved. If you scored very much better than the average, chances are you're already engaged in fitness training or have a highly active life-style.

Caution

Stop the test *immediately* if you experience any symptoms of overexertion—dizziness, nausea, weakness, shortness of breath, or chest pain. Sit down, recover, and consult a doctor.

Weight

Because fitness is related to weight, you'll want to compare your weight with the range for your age, height, and sex. If you're seriously over or under the average weight reading, you may have a medical problem and should consult a doctor, especially if you're considering a fitness program.

Use these charts to determine how your present weight compares with the most desirable weight for your height and build. Measure your height in your bare feet.

	Men				Women		
Height	Small build	Medium build	Large build	Height	Small build	Medium build	Large build
	(±4%)	(±5%)	(±6%)		(±4%)	(±5%)	(±6%)
5' 2"	123	131	138	4' 9"	107	114	122
3"	127	135	143	10"	109	116	124
4"	131	139	147	11"	111	118	126
5"	134	142	151	5' 0"	114	121	129
6"	138	146	155	1"	117	124	132
7"	141	150	159	2"	120	128	136
8"	145	154	163	3"	123	131	139
9"	149	158	168	4"	127	135	144
10"	154	162	172	5"	131	139	148
11"	158	167	177	6"	134	142	151
6' 0"	163	172	182	7"	138	146	155
1"	169	177	187	8"	141	150	159
2"	174	182	192	9"	145	153	162

Flexibility and strength

Flexibility and strength are really only fitness measures insofar as they affect posture and your ability to accomplish everyday tasks easily. Improperly exercised or inactive muscles tire quickly. Common symptoms are aches and pains, particularly in the back. If you restrict your activity because of poor muscle tone and endurance, then your fitness needs improvement in strength and flexibility.

Not too long ago exercise physiologists believed that everyone should be able to perform a certain number of push-ups, or sit-ups, or jumping jacks within a given time. Such tests do set a standard of strength and endurance—you may find that working up to these levels gives you fitness to enjoy the activities in your life. But the choice is yours. *You* must de-

Flexibility tests

Try these four simple tests to determine your present flexibility.

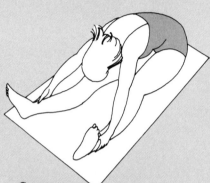

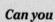

Can you
• reach your ankles when sitting with legs out in front of you?

Can you
• move each arm from straight in front of you to 45 degrees behind?

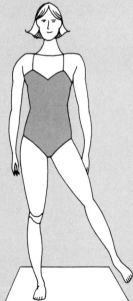

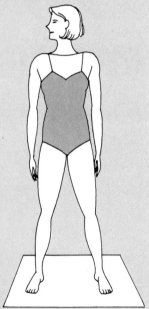

Can you
• lift each leg 45 degrees straight out to the side when standing?

Can you
• turn your neck 90 degrees to either side?

Some other pulse figures

Your pulse at rest and at peak activity also measures your fitness. But it's quite difficult to work with such numbers. Mood, time of day, age, medication, drinking coffee—many things influence your resting pulse. You'll find, on average, that your resting pulse becomes slower as your fitness increases. Similarly, increasing fitness means your heart beats at lower rates during exertion.

While exercising you'll generally want to maintain a certain pulse range of maximum benefit. This is a way of checking your body's output level. After a few weeks of training, you'll know when you've reached the target effort range, and you won't need to refer very often to your pulse.

cide how much strength training is appropriate for you and what muscle groups deserve special attention.

How to exercise

Before you get started on your own exercise program, you'll need some basic rules. Whether you're a cyclist, a skater, a rower, or a table tennis champion in training, follow these general principles of exercise—most of them are just common sense.

• Start any exercise program with modest exertion and work up *gradually*. A week at each beginning step is often recommended. You can't become fit overnight —beneficial effects become measurable in about 3 weeks and significant at 3 to 6 months.

Health worries and too-often-postponed good fitness intentions can push people into crash exercising. This merely translates a mental crisis into what can become a physical crisis. Don't commit this mistake.

• Regularity is in many ways the most important exercise rule. A sporadic workout every 3 weeks or so is not only insufficient, it could be dangerous, particularly as you get older. Sudden sustained exercise is dangerous to an underprepared, unfit body. The sooner it's over the better.

Regular exercise both creates and *maintains* fitness, even at levels of 30 minutes 2 to 3 times per week.

• Don't exercise beyond the limits of your doctor's advice.

• *Never* exercise when you suffer from an infection. Bacterial and viral infections are apt to worsen with exercise.

Take it easy if you've been bedridden for a while. After 3 weeks off your feet, your exercise capacity will have diminished 30 percent or more. Don't expect to perform right away at your previous levels.

• Make a habit of performing appropriate warm-up exercises before vigorous activity. And cool down gradually when you've finished your workout; walk around for a few minutes before you sit down.

• On some days you'll exercise more intensively than others. Trying to push back your limits every time you work out is wrongheaded. No one's body is equally capable and willing each day—and it'll let you know when the effort is too much.

Recognizing and treating frostbite

Frostbite is a serious injury; you must get out of the cold and treat a suspected frostbite as quickly as possible. You'll recognize frostbite as a hard, white patch on exposed or insufficiently protected skin (hands, face, and feet are the most commonly affected areas). Frostbitten tissue is dead; there's not much you can do about that, but you do want to limit the damage and revive nearby threatened tissue.

Soak a suspected frostbite in lukewarm water, between 100 and 104 degrees F.—you can use an ordinary fever thermometer to check the water's temperature. It's important that the water not be above 109 degrees, which would further damage the frostbitten area. Never rub snow on a frostbitten extremity—it just makes the problem worse.

Exercise and hot weather

80°–84° F.—be careful, watch out for signs of fatigue

85°–88° F.—don't do anything strenuous

89° F. and above—don't exercise at all

• Exercise is okay at any time of day. Dawn is fine, so are the moments before you retire for the night—whatever suits you and makes it easier for you to stick with an exercise routine.

• Stop exercising immediately if you experience any of the following symptoms of overexertion:

> chest pressure or pain
> shortness of breath
> dizziness
> weakness
> nausea

Soreness, tenderness, or swelling are clear signs of injury. Stop exercising and find out what's wrong. Chances are very good you'll worsen any injury if you ignore your body's warnings.

• When you're physically active out-of-doors, always take temperatures into account. In cold weather, check the windchill factor. Equivalent windchill temperatures measure how quickly you can become frostbitten. Wear protective clothing, particularly around your head and face, if you're exercising in the lower range of safe temperature.

Hot weather brings the risk of heat exhaustion and heatstroke. Be alert for the first symptoms of either. (Salt tablets—not recommended—don't necessarily protect you.) At the high end of the safe temperature zone, wear the lightest possible clothing. Allow yourself a week to adjust to hot weather if you've traveled to a warmer climate—workouts must initially be somewhat lighter than at lower temperatures.

No one ever becomes 100 percent acclimated to a great change in altitude. Three weeks at high altitude restores much of your performance level, but you'll never reach your low-altitude peak. Remember, your body can't create oxygen, and less of it is available at higher altitudes.

• Think about your equipment: clothing should not restrict movement; the wrong shoes can cause injury; protective gear must be intact.

Now that you're acquainted with the rules of exercise, we can get down to business, starting, of course, with suggestions for your warm-up.

What windchill is all about

Our concept of *windchill factor* dates from some 1941 experiments conducted in the Antarctic. Scientists timed the freezing of a half pint of water under varying conditions of temperature and wind speed. The higher the wind speed, the faster heat is carried away from a beaker of water, or from a human body (our bodies are about the same density as water, and composed mostly of water).

Windchill temperatures are the best way of measuring actual weather effects on your body. In the colder seasons, listen for windchill information in weather broadcasts or calculate it for yourself from the table below.

Windchill factor chart

Estimated wind speed (in mph)	Actual thermometer reading (in degrees Fahrenheit)							
	50°F	40°F	30°F	20°F	10°F	0°F	−10°F	−20°F
	Equivalent temperature							
Calm	50	40	30	20	10	0	−10	−20
5	48	37	27	16	6	−5	−15	−26
10	40	28	16	4	−9	−24	−33	−46
15	36	22	9	−5	−18	−32	−45	−58
20	32	18	4	−10	−25	−39	−53	−67
25	30	16	0	−15	−29	−44	−59	−74
30	28	13	−2	−18	−33	−48	−63	−79
35	27	11	−4	−20	−35	−51	−67	−82
40	26	10	−6	−21	−37	−53	−69	−85

Wind speeds greater than 40 mph have little additional effect.

☐ INCREASING DANGER
Danger from freezing of exposed flesh.
■ GREAT DANGER
For all temperatures below 50° F., dress warmly and stay dry.

5

Choosing an exercise

Why you should always warm up

There are sound physiological reasons for your warm-up: every degree centigrade you raise an inactive muscle's temperature brings up your cells' energy production (metabolism) about 13 percent. After a 5- to 15-minute warm-up, your muscles are near their ideal working temperature. Equally important, your warm-up raises your circulation and heart activity more smoothly to higher levels.

Before you start any kind of demanding physical activity, you'll want to warm up—loosen up your body and raise your muscles' temperature. Not only does a warm-up improve your performance, but it'll also lessen the possibility of muscle strain or ligament damage (injury). A warm-up, however, isn't just physical conditioning, it's also psychological. Warm-up focuses your mind on the activities ahead and dispels tension.

You'll be wise to start every exercise session with at least 5 to 15 minutes of light calisthenics and stretching. Then begin your exercises gradually. This reasoning applies also to heavy chores around the house or yard. Warm up before attempting to shovel snow or move heavy furniture.

General and specific warm-up

You should choose your warm-up exercises from two categories: general stretches and movements for your whole body, and more specific actions mimicking the sport or activity you're preparing for. If you're about to play baseball, for example, throw the ball easily for a while, warming up gradually to full power. Joggers and cyclists alike benefit from loosely running in place for a few moments. Tennis players swing the racket arm in long arcs, soccer players kick phantom balls, high divers may bend and stretch their torsos.

Whatever the specific movements you choose for your warm-up, combine them with five or six of the basic warm-up exercises shown here. In general a 5- to 10-minute warm-up is all you'll need—but don't wait more than 20 or 30 minutes after warming up to begin activity in earnest.

Cool down

When you're through exercising, your body needs to return circulation and metabolism to nonexercising levels. You can make this a smooth transition by "cooling down" properly. Walk around for 5 minutes or so after your workout or do light calisthenics and stretching. No need to bundle yourself in extra clothing, but add another garment if you feel cold.

Stretch with patience

In stretching, especially in warming up and cooling down, more isn't better. Just extend the muscle until you feel tightness. Then hold it. Don't jiggle, bounce, push, or otherwise try to massage the stretched muscle. Leave it alone. If you feel any discomfort, do less. The watchward for these exercises is patience.

Flexibility

Along with endurance and strength, flexibility is one of your three fundamental fitness goals. It's also slow to develop, so don't try to stretch too far too soon.

Ideas about flexibility training have changed somewhat over the last few decades. For one thing, not every exercise that pulls something in your body is necessarily a good one. Some stretches pit a large muscle against a smaller one. In heel raises, for example, a large muscle (triceps surae) behind the heel can overstretch smaller sole muscles (plantar muscles) and damage ligaments. Although this exercise was once prescribed for strengthening arches, it actually weakens the arch.

Stretching a muscle is certainly a good thing, but not if the muscle is actually torn or stretched so far that it can no longer contract properly. Such unwanted stretching can occur, too, if you put your body into a posture that allows large muscles to pull your back out of line. This can happen in straight-legged sit-ups and leg-lifts done from a lying-down-on-your-back position: your large hip muscles (the iliopsoas), which can pull with a force of 1,300 pounds or more, do most of the work in these exercises. Their strength easily overpowers the many smaller muscles of the lower back, causing a pronounced inward curvature of the spine. With a little modification—bent knees, to keep your lower back firmly on the floor, or turning on your side—these exercises become helpful ones.

The proper way to perform any stretch is to extend yourself until you feel tightness, that first pull. Hold it, wait a few seconds, and stretch a little farther, until you feel another pull. Your body will send pain signals if you're about to exceed your limits. Don't ignore the warnings. Pain isn't a positive exercise measure. Bouncing at the utmost extent of any stretch (a "ballistic" stretch) causes pain, just as it causes damage to your body. Tiny ligament or muscle tears can easily happen when you insist on stretching "till it hurts."

The exercises presented here will improve your flexibility. Do them slowly and do them regularly. You can expect noticeably greater suppleness within 5 or 6 weeks.

Strength

Exercising for strength doesn't mean that you'll need to buy a set of weights and special belts to hold your-

(continued on page 51)

Warm-up exercises

Start every exercise session with at least five minutes of light calisthentics and stretching. These eight exercises will warm up your major muscle groups, but you can substitute any favorites of your choice.

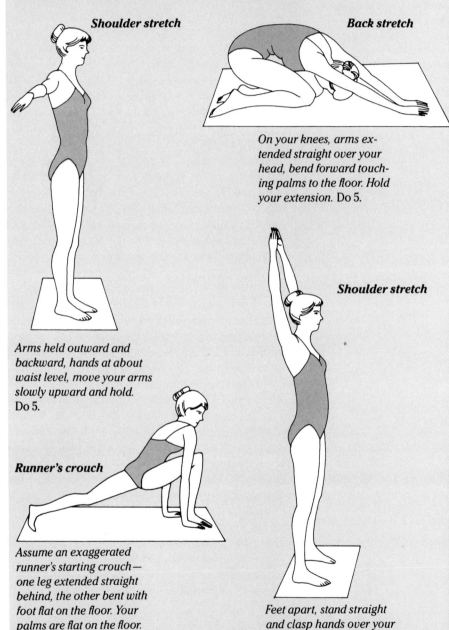

Shoulder stretch

Back stretch

On your knees, arms extended straight over your head, bend forward touching palms to the floor. Hold your extension. Do 5.

Shoulder stretch

Arms held outward and backward, hands at about waist level, move your arms slowly upward and hold. Do 5.

Runner's crouch

Assume an exaggerated runner's starting crouch — one leg extended straight behind, the other bent with foot flat on the floor. Your palms are flat on the floor. Hold and reverse the position, being careful not to bounce. Do 5.

Feet apart, stand straight and clasp hands over your head. Pull your shoulders backward, keeping arms high. Hold and relax. Do 5.

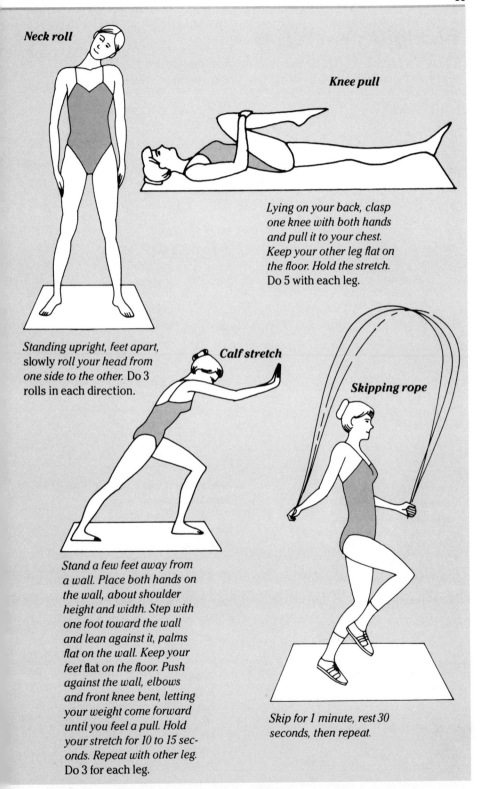

Neck roll

Knee pull

Lying on your back, clasp one knee with both hands and pull it to your chest. Keep your other leg flat on the floor. Hold the stretch. Do 5 with each leg.

Standing upright, feet apart, slowly *roll your head from one side to the other.* Do 3 rolls in each direction.

Calf stretch

Skipping rope

Stand a few feet away from a wall. Place both hands on the wall, about shoulder height and width. Step with one foot toward the wall and lean against it, palms flat on the wall. Keep your feet flat on the floor. Push against the wall, elbows and front knee bent, letting your weight come forward until you feel a pull. Hold your stretch for 10 to 15 seconds. Repeat with other leg. Do 3 for each leg.

Skip for 1 minute, rest 30 seconds, then repeat.

Flexibility exercises

These six exercises help extend your range of motion. Do them slowly and you'll stretch at the same time. Do each exercise five times.

Side stretch

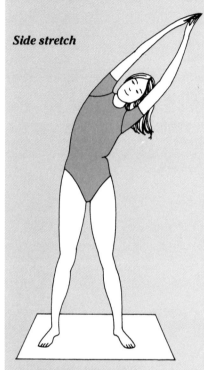

Flexed-knee toe touch

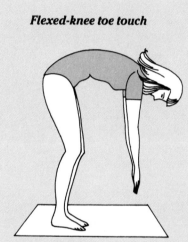

With hands clasped above your head and legs apart, bend slowly from the waist, first to one side and then the other. Hold each stretch for a few seconds.

Bend forward, knees slightly flexed. Stop when you feel the tug of muscles behind the leg. Let gravity gently stretch you farther downward. If you don't reach the floor at first, that's okay. Don't strain and, above all, don't bounce while stretching.

Judo split

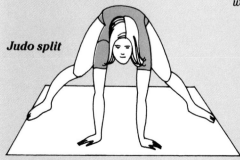

Bend over and put your palms on the floor for support. With knees straight, spread your legs as far apart as they'll go. Hold your stretch for a few seconds.

Reach

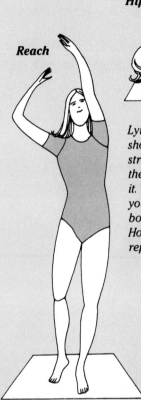

Hip pull

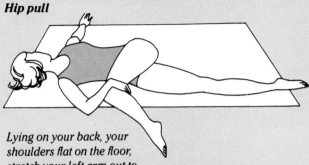

Lying on your back, your shoulders flat on the floor, stretch your left arm out to the side and turn to look at it. With your right arm pull your left leg across your body as far as possible. Hold for 10 seconds and repeat for the right leg.

Imagine you're trying to touch the ceiling, first with one arm and then the other. Get up on tiptoe; reach as high as you can and hold it.

Side twist

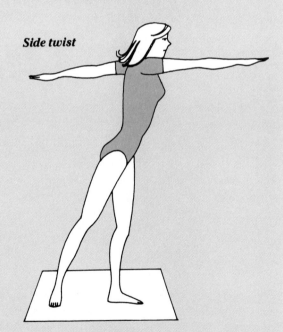

Feet apart, arms extended and palms down, turn slowly to one side as far as you can. Hold and turn to the other side.

Strength exercises

These eleven exercises will increase your strength quickly and with little risk because they use your body weight only. You should repeat strength exercises as many times as you can. Move on to a more difficult exercise when one begins to feel too easy.

Back leg raise

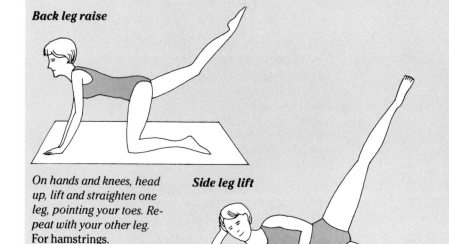

On hands and knees, head up, lift and straighten one leg, pointing your toes. Repeat with your other leg. For hamstrings.

Side leg lift

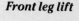

Lying on your side, head propped on one arm, lift your free leg upward. Turn onto your other side and repeat with your other leg. For thigh muscles.

Front leg lift

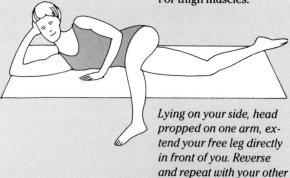

Lying on your side, head propped on one arm, extend your free leg directly in front of you. Reverse and repeat with your other leg. For thigh muscles and buttocks.

Half push-up

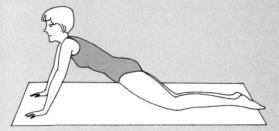

Easier than a full push-up.
With your hands outside
your shoulders, raise yourself up with your arms,
keeping bent knees in contact with the floor. For triceps, pectorals, and
shoulder muscles.

Push-up

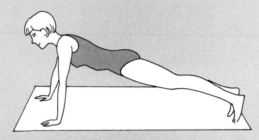

Keep your back straight,
weight on your toes, hands
outside your shoulders, and
raise yourself. Almost, but
not quite, touch the floor
with your chest on the way
down. For triceps, pecto-
rals, shoulder, and abdominal muscles.

Curl-up

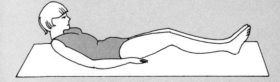

Lying on your back, knees
slightly bent, hands at your
sides, curl your head and
shoulders off the floor,
keeping your chin tucked
on your chest. Curl-ups
are an easier form of sit-
ups. For hip and abdominal
muscles.

(continued on page 44)

Strength exercises —Continued

V-up

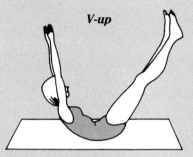

Twisting sit-up

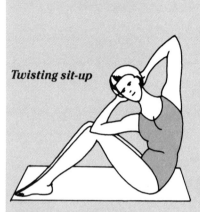

A superior kind of sit-up, but harder to perform. Lying on your back, arms extended behind your head, legs straight, bring your arms and legs up at the same time, forming a V with your body. For hip and abdominal muscles.

Lying on your back, knees well bent and hands clasped behind your head, raise yourself and try to touch one elbow to the opposite knee. Alternate twists, first left elbow to right knee, then the reverse. For hip and abdominal muscles.

Hip raise

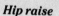

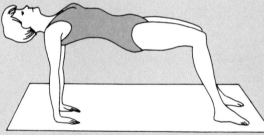

Half knee bend

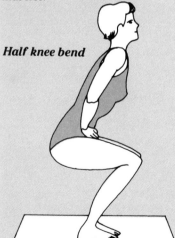

From a sitting position, place your palms on the floor behind you and raise your hips off the floor until your body is horizontal. For back muscles.

Back lift

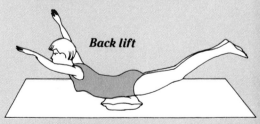

Feet apart, hands on your hips, squat until thighs are horizontal, but go no deeper, and return to upright. For buttocks and quadriceps.

Lying facedown, with a firm cushion under your hips and stomach, lift your head, arms, and legs off the floor. You may keep your arms at your sides or extended beyond your head (more difficult). Just lift, don't arch backward. For back muscles and hamstrings.

Weight-training exercises

These seven weight-training exercises build and toughen muscles.

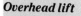

Overhead lift

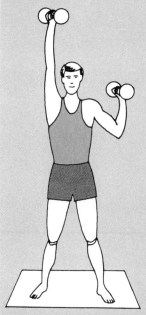

Side lift

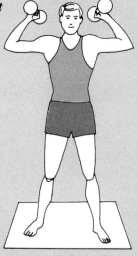

Holding dumbbells at shoulder level, extend both dumbbells straight out to the sides; flex your arms and bend your elbows to bring them back. For shoulder and upper back muscles.

Lift one dumbbell straight up above your head; lower it to shoulder level, and raise the other. For triceps, pectorals, and shoulder muscles.

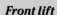

Front lift

With dumbbells held in front of you against your chest, extend them ahead of you and flex your arms to bring them back. For pectorals, shoulder, upper back, and upper side muscles.

(continued on page 46)

Weight-training exercises —Continued

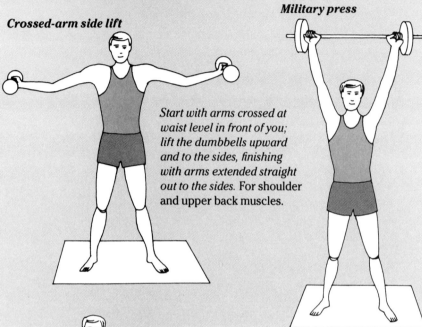

Crossed-arm side lift

Start with arms crossed at waist level in front of you; lift the dumbbells upward and to the sides, finishing with arms extended straight out to the sides. For shoulder and upper back muscles.

Military press

Feet apart, gripping the barbell palms outward, lift the weight straight overhead until your elbows are straight. For triceps, pectorals, and shoulder muscles

Curls

Feet apart, with the barbell hanging at arms' length, flex your biceps to lift the weight to shoulder level. Keep your elbows in to your side; hands are palms outward when gripping the weight at thigh level. For biceps and forearm muscles.

Bench Press

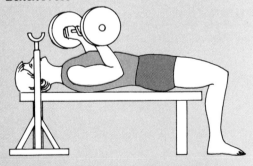

Lying on a bench, feet on the floor, grip the barbell palms outward and lift it off its overhead supports. (Your bench must be equipped with supports to perform this exercise.) Lower the weight to your chest, then lift straight up. For pectorals (especially good) and shoulder muscles.

Posture exercises

Posture exercises mix balance and relaxation. These twelve exercises will improve your posture while improving flexibility.

Neck pull

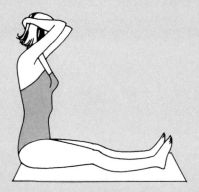

Straight-arm circles

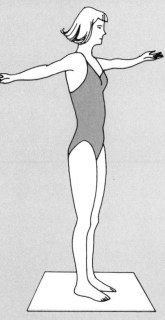

Seated with your legs extended straight out in front of you and your hands clasped behind your head, pull forward with the arms, push backward with your head. Do 3, 10 seconds each. Develops neck strength; helps you hold your head erect.

Supine reach

Lying on your back, knees bent and feet flat on the floor, move your arms, palms up, from your sides to a position horizontally over your head. Then bring your arms back to your sides. Do 10. Eases protruding shoulders.

Standing with your arms extended out to your sides, palms up, make slow circles with straight arms. Do for 1 minute or more. Straightens shoulders.

(continued on page 48)

Posture exercises —Continued

Dowel stretch

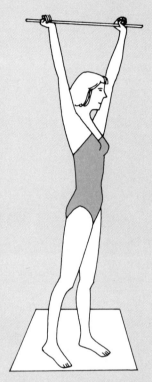

Straight-arm suspension

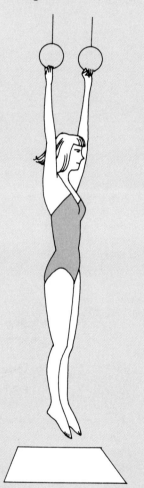

*Standing upright, feet apart,
grasp a dowel or broom
handle in both hands. Bring
the dowel slowly over your
head and as far back as you
can—but keep your back as
straight as possible. Do 5.
Straightens shoulders.*

*Hang straight-armed from a
bar or gym rings. Hang for
15 seconds to 1 minute— as
long as you can—twice.
Straightens lower back and
shoulders.*

Circular shrug

Hula

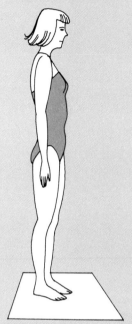

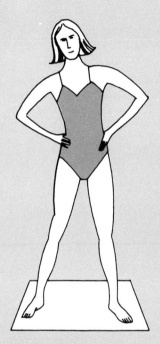

Standing, arms at your
sides, shrug your shoulders
in circles. Do for at least 1
minute. *Corrects drooping
shoulders.*

With hands on your hips,
slowly rotate your pelvis as
though using a hula hoop.
*(Using a hula hoop will
probably make you swivel
too quickly.)* Reverse direction from time to time. Do
for 2 minutes. *Reduces
lower back curve.*

Hip bend

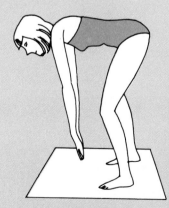

Let your arms hang loosely
and bend forward from the
hips. Keeping your back
straight, bob a little in your
bent position. Do 5.
Straightens lower back.

(continued on page 50)

Posture exercises —Continued

Trunk straightener

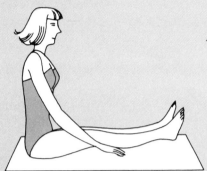

Back stretch

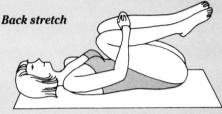

Sit on the floor with your legs straight out in front of you. Now, hold your back and head perfectly erect. Relax after 10 or 15 seconds and repeat. Do 5; breathe naturally while sitting erect. *Reduces back curvature.*

Lying on your back, draw your knees tightly up to your chest and clasp your hands around them. Hold your position for 1 minute. Do 2. *Evens out a back tilt to one side or the other.*

Toe crawl

Sitting, knees well bent and with feet flat on the floor, draw a towel toward you with your toes—use small curling toe movements without letting the heel or ball of your foot leave the floor. Stop when your toes feel tight and tired. *Strengthens arches; recommended for flat feet.*

Shoulder lift

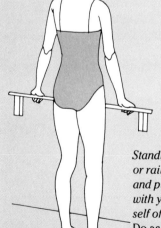

Standing at a hip-high bar or rail, put hands on bar and push against the bar with your palms. Lift yourself off the floor if you can. Do as many as you can. *Straightens upper back.*

Don't hold your breath

In exercising for strength, or in any other exertion, don't hold your breath during effort. Holding your breath and taking on a load makes your heart's job very difficult.

Strength *continued*

self together while you groan under a cruel mass of iron. A high fitness level demands muscles that accept loads easily, that recover quickly—muscles that enable you to participate fully in whatever physical activities you think you might enjoy. It may be your choice, of course, to build your muscles to their fullest potential. Body building is now recognized as a major sport. The strength exercises recommended here, however, serve a more general fitness purpose.

You'll probably be surprised at how fast muscles develop. A daily workout shows results in as little as 1 week.

Overload

The first principle of strength training—basic also to endurance and flexibility training—is overload. You must tax your muscles in each workout with just a little more effort than is comfortable. As in many other aspects of our lives, the qualities we hope to develop in ourselves can grow only through effort. However, don't push yourself to the point of diminishing return, the threshold of overintensity, of overstress. Work your muscles hard, but stop when you become tired. Never ignore muscle pain; the sharp sensation of a muscle pull or tear means that you've gone too far.

Repetition

The second principle in strength training is repetition. Muscles needn't only to grow, as an overload helps them to do, but to become more efficient. A repetitious cycle of muscular contraction and relaxation builds endurance. That's why strength exercises seem always to come in sets of 5, 10, 20, or more.

If you stick with a training program, your muscles' improved staying power can become something of an embarrassment. You'll notice a 20-minute workout that once brought protest from your muscles soon isn't even getting them properly warmed up. You're no longer overloading them. Maybe a 30- or 40-minute workout is needed. If you don't want to lengthen your exercise period, then do more demanding exercises within your allotted time. Muscles that aren't really challenged stop improving.

One final word: in exercising for strength, or in any other exertion, *don't* hold your breath during effort. Holding your breath and taking on a load makes your heart's job very difficult.

What and when to drink

Water is the best hydrating fluid. Your body absorbs it faster than other fluids. Drink before and after exercise, and if your workout continues for longer than 45 minutes, drink during exercise as well.

Antagonistic muscles

Antagonistic muscles do not, as their name might suggest, hamper one another. They work in a very balanced relationship. One group relaxes while the antagonistic (opposite) group contracts. This action explains how you can, for example, bend from the waist either frontward or backward.

Working with dumbbells and barbells

Fitness certainly doesn't require weight training, but if you're pretty fit already and want to try it, go ahead. A little lifting isn't a bad idea. Athletes in most sports train to some degree with weights. It toughens the muscles—cutting down on injuries—and can raise their anaerobic, peak-load, power.

The chief training measurement with weights is the repetition maximum (RM), the greatest weight you can lift a specific number of times. For example, if you can raise a 60-pound weight over your head 10 times, you have 10 RM at that weight and for that particular lift. Ten RM is a convenient muscle-building level, so you might work to get your 10 RM up to 70 pounds and higher (rather than stick with 60 pounds and have to do more repetitions than 10).

Only the most basic lifts are shown here. Many lifts can place underdeveloped muscles and unprotected joints in real jeopardy. Don't attempt heavy lifts or more advanced exercises without the assistance and advice of a knowledgeable trainer.

Posture

Perhaps you've never thought about it, but our ability to stand upright is an engineering miracle. Balance is one necessary part of the accomplishment. Sensors in your inner ear provide tilt information in the form of signals to your brain. These signals, along with touch sensations and visual cues, are processed by your brain into muscle commands. And that brings us to the second necessity for standing upright: a muscle arrangement that defies gravity.

Your body acts a little like a television mast, held upright by equally tensioned guy wires. Except in your body the guy wires are muscles, pulling with adjustable tension down the front and down the back of your frame. Generally speaking, for every muscle group that acts to bend you forward another muscle group in your neck, back, thigh, or calf acts to bend you backward. If your muscle groups' pull is nicely balanced, you'll have a comfortable upright posture. This is an example of how antagonistic muscle groups work. Antagonists pull lightly against each other, maintaining posture, until a particular flex or motion is desired. Then one group relaxes while the opposing group is allowed to contract more powerfully.

Posture problems can arise when opposing muscle

groups become too tense, pulling harder than is necessary against each other. You may have experienced muscle "knots" in your neck and shoulders as a result of this tension. A more serious problem arises when one antagonist loses strength or flexibility—a muscle, ideally, must be able to contract powerfully, but also to relax and stretch when its antagonist is pulling the other way. When your muscles work poorly together, usually because they aren't exercised enough, you may suffer from pronounced spine curvature, sway back, slumped shoulders, a drooping head, and pain in the lower back and shoulders. True, diseases of bone, muscle, and organs can cause low back pain, but doctors say that 80 percent of low back pain arises from unconditioned muscles.

The dangers of overstretching

Just as flabby, unconditioned muscles contribute to posture problems, so do overstretched ligaments and tendons. The many small muscles holding your spine erect are attached to your ribs with many small tendons. You should keep them all flexible, but never overdo it. About the worst thing you can do, once having eased yourself into a good supple stretch, is to start bouncing and bobbing for that extra little pull. You're already at the limits of what your musculature can handle. Very likely your added bounce will succeed in tearing or hyperextending something.

Posture exercises

Any well-rounded group of calisthenics, and exercise such as walking, contributes to good posture. For more specific posture problems, some special exercises are provided here. Remember, exercise can strengthen your muscles, but good posture also requires muscular relaxation. We convert much everyday stress into muscle tension, carrying unresolved conflict stored in our knotted muscles. Almost any kind of exercise can help, sometimes dramatically, to dispel such tension.

Your exercise program

Here are some hints for putting together your own exercise program:

• **Checkup.** Have a checkup if you're over age 35 or have any kind of medical problem.

• **Warm-up and cool down.** Choose three or four exercises for your warm-up. Vary them from session to session; not only is variety in warm-up more interesting, you're less likely to neglect a needed stretch. Always count on cooling down for 5 minutes. Just walk around for a while or perform light calisthenics.

• **Activities.** Do what you enjoy most. Vigorous, aerobic activity needn't occupy you for more than 20 to 30 minutes, three times a week. (After you've reached a higher level of aerobic fitness—after 5 to 6 months—two workouts per week will maintain fitness.)

Have fun

You needn't suffer to keep fit. Your exercise program should include activities you enjoy, whether they're team sports or exercises you perform alone. Your exercise time is personal time. Enjoy yourself while being good to your body.

• **Endurance.** When you train for fitness, it's the first few minutes of exertion that count most. That's why interval training works so well to condition you. For people already in fit shape, it's the last few minutes of effort that expand endurance—but that doesn't mean athletes are fitter, only that they can perform at a higher level. There's no extra benefit for you in more intense, competitive training if athletic performance isn't one of your personal goals. Whatever your training goals, avoid exhaustion.

• **Measuring progress.** Undoubtedly, your physical condition will improve with exercise, and you'll notice it—in your sleep, energy level, outlook, appetite, and more. If you'd like to keep track of your improvements in a more concrete way, keep records: an exercise diary illustrates your progress toward higher work capacity; a pulse record, taken at rest from time to time, certifies greater heart and circulatory power; and a few periodic tape measurements around the waist, thighs, chest, calves, biceps, etc., keep track of where you're losing inches and gaining them (it's easiest to have someone assist you with the tape—more honest, too). Don't forget to log your weight.

• **Above all, *stay* fit.** Try some sports and activities you think you might enjoy. Evaluate your average day for fitness: do you walk much? Are you on your feet for at least two hours? A close look at the way you live and work will almost certainly disclose pleasurable opportunities to combine a little effort with your daily tasks. Physical activities that become habitual are your goal.

Helpful checklist

Use this checklist to see you through each workout session until you're into a routine.

☐ Ten minutes of warm-up

☐ Twenty minutes of exercise that maintains your 10-second pulse between 70% and 85% of your maximum heart rate (see chart on inside front cover)

☐ Five minutes of cool-down

☐ Weekly records of exercise, including the activity, its duration, your maintained pulse, and the exercise's purpose—to build endurance, strength, or flexibility. You might want to use this form:

Date	Exercise	Maintained pulse	Purpose	Weight

6

Aerobic activity

How you can evaluate aerobic activities
With the best aerobic exercises, you'll exercise large muscle groups in more or less continuous motion. Then your heart can reach an appropriate exertion level and remain there for the duration of the exercise. By this standard, volleyball, for example, isn't quite as constant as swimming.

From a spectator's viewpoint, most sports look like short bursts of work separated by longish pauses in the action. Because the inactive intervals in football or baseball, for example, are so long in comparison to actual play, we can't even say that such pastimes much resemble aerobic interval training. That doesn't mean that team sports and other broken activities don't have an aerobic benefit—they do, but much less than the best aerobic exercises.

Those activities at the top of the aerobic heap generally involve propelling yourself around in one way or another—bicycling, cross-country skiing, dancing, jogging, rowing, swimming, and walking. This isn't surprising: a high aerobic value means that your body's large muscle groups are kept in more or less continuous use. Working the large muscles at a steady rate builds heart, lung, and circulatory power. That's why nearly all athletes, in every sport, place training emphasis on aerobic conditioning.

Considered from another angle, however, aerobics, too, has a few shortcomings. Just as exercising for high strength does little for your aerobic capacity, most aerobic exercise requires little flexibility. Rhythmic, repetitive muscle motions need to be supplemented with stretches. You'll find you suffer fewer pulls and strains as a result.

Before you begin any of these aerobic activities, be sure to review chapters 2 and 4, "Health, fitness, and exercise" and "Getting ready." They contain important guidelines for achieving good training effect and exercising safely.

Bicycling

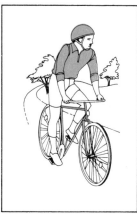

Bicycling doesn't stress joints vulnerable to injury; it's safe and effective. Practically anyone—even someone overweight—can enjoy cycling.

Bicycling
If you're looking for a first-rate aerobic activity and can get away from heavy city traffic, bicycling can be a beautiful, healthful experience. It is also especially good exercise for those who are overweight, having the advantage of keeping weight off vulnerable joints. As with other activities, start slowly. The large leg muscles must be conditioned gradually, since they're doing all the work. Your pulse rate and muscles' fatigue will let you know when enough is enough.

In the right kind of terrain, working uphill, resting on the down slope, cycling has the aerobic efficiency of interval training. On level stretches you can sprint, cruise, or just enjoy the scenery—it's all aerobic. With bicycles, however, you'll need to make some important equipment choices and practice safety.

Equipment

First of all, a light, well-made touring bike is versatile. Five gears suffice for the casual cyclist; that's about as many gears as ever get used on most ten-speed bikes. Racing handlebars, though popular, have several drawbacks. If you're not a racer, you'll probably want to sit upright and look around when cycling. Most racing-bike owners sit up anyway, holding directly onto the metal handlebars, closer in to the bike's steering post. Wrists absorb more vibration here, and there are no protective rubber grips to facilitate bike handling. The laws of physics—the same generous laws that can make a tipsy, two-wheeler stable as long as you keep pedaling—reduce your steering control as you move your hands closer and closer to the steering post. It makes very little sense to buy equipment that you *intend* to use improperly, so carefully examine your needs before making a purchase. (A racing saddle, by the way, is designed for the bent, racing position.)

Exercise

As much fun as cycling can be, no aerobic exercise has less value for flexibility. Make sure your personal program includes a full range of stretches and strength exercises for your upper body—muscles never used in cycling.

Safety

Wear a bicycle helmet. Bicyclists fall down for a number of reasons, most of them unexpected; you don't want to take the full impact on your head.

Shoes with heels slip off the pedals less often than smooth soles. Get pedal straps, if you wish, but they're a nuisance in stop-and-go riding and an entanglement in spills.

Accident statistics make it clear that bicycling in traffic is dangerous. Try to locate more secluded routes for yourself or use bike trails where available. At night, use lights and reflectors, front, rear, and on your pedals, wheels, and clothes.

Bicycles don't work well on wet surfaces, particu-

Learning to spin

Cadence is the number of revolutions per minute (rpm) that you turn a bicycle's pedals. Your aim should be to maintain a constant high number of rpms without wearing yourself out. This is generally accomplished by pedaling rapidly in low gears. Cyclists call this spinning. Once you've mastered spinning, you'll be able to travel long distances without tiring.

The average rider usually pedals fewer than 40 rpms. An accomplished cyclist will have a cadence of 90 to 120 rpms. You can determine your rpms by timing yourself for a minute while you pedal on level ground. Count the number of times your right knee rises.

Using a low gear will make it possible to maintain a rapid cadence. Each higher gear reduces the number of pedal revolutions per minute.

Exercise bikes

If riding a bicycle outdoors is impractical, try an exercise bike. If you have a weight problem, for example, pedaling on an exercise bike won't put extra strain on your back and knees, and you'll get all the benefits of an aerobic exercise.

larly during braking. Loose gravel or sand is another braking hazard. On any surface, apply your rear brake before squeezing the front brake. Otherwise the rear wheel tries to come forward, usually turning the bike sideways.

Indoor cycling

Because cycling is best limited to fair weather and daylight hours, you may enjoy it as a supplement or alternate to your other regular activities. But you can still cycle any time of day and in weather that makes even walking or jogging impossible—you can if you invest in a stationary bicycle apparatus—an exercycle. Most come equipped with timers, speedometers, or other devices to measure effort level, and tension adjustments to increase the load. As with other activities, your goal is a 20- to 30-minute workout three times a week.

Exercise bikes are usually parked in front of TV sets, where indoor cyclists catch a soap opera or the evening news while keeping up a high aerobic fitness level. Or, to read your exercise time away, purchase any of the book racks now available to mount on your handlebars.

Cross-country skiing

Cross-country skiing, also called Nordic skiing, can require extremely intense effort. As with jogging, you must condition yourself as a preliminary to beginning this sport. But Nordic skiing exercises more muscle groups than jogging and without the pounding contact of running. Of course, cross-country skiing doesn't have to be so strenuous. On level, packed snow, walking or skiing at about 3 miles an hour takes the same energy. (The skiers actually feel less fatigued than the walkers, because skiers divide the work between arm and leg muscles!) Skiing faster or skiing uphill is another story. No other activity calls for such sustained aerobic power. And the air you're breathing is always cold. Asthmatics shouldn't try this activity. Heart patients, even in good condition, need a doctor's okay for cross-country skiing. It's usually not recommended.

Because we still think of downhill skiing (Alpine skiing) first when someone mentions skiing, we also think immediately of expense. Cross-country uses less costly, less specialized equipment. You won't have to journey to a distant ski run—any snowy landscape will do—and you won't have to pay for ski-lift passes, ei-

Cross-country skiing

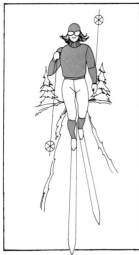

Depending on your condition and inclination toward exertion, cross-country skiing can be an invigorating aerobic workout or as relaxing as a brisk walk.

Dancing as exercise

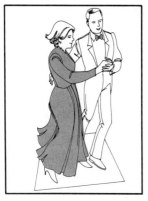

Maybe you don't think of dancing as an exercise, but it becomes one if you just keep going without interruption at more or less the same pace for 20 minutes. If some numbers have slower beats, just add a few extra minutes to your session.

ther. So cross-country skiing is not expensive. It's limited to the winter season, however, and you'll have to find other fitness activities for the warmer weather.

Significant injuries in cross-country skiing usually happen on the down slope. Loss of control, icy patches, and unnoticed obstructions are always downhill hazards. More commonly, beginners hurt themselves by overexertion. So many muscles are in use, a new skier may become completely exhausted before sensing what's happened. Explore your limits cautiously in this activity.

Dancing

All the best aerobic features are built into ballet and modern dance. Warm-up and stretching are always part of the training routine. And ballet has refined its exercises with the practical knowledge of several hundred years' experience. Newer dance styles have borrowed from ballet. The results are vigorous aerobic exercises. Classical dance styles don't monopolize fitness, however; tap dancing, disco, clog dancing, square dance, and other folk dances can be just as healthful when combined with a good warm-up and preliminary stretch.

Because dance can be as enjoyable at slower tempos as at accelerated beats, the beginning stages are never boring—dance often requires the participation of your mind as well as your body; imagination, too, is a working asset in dance. There's always something to learn, a new variation to try. Professional dancers never stop learning, nor do they stop training. Fitness tests usually find ballet dancers score higher than other athletes. Of course, you needn't have this professional obsession with training to achieve important fitness goals. Thirty to 40 minutes three times a week suffices.

Some dance training—jazz dancing, for example— has less conditioning effect. Mix your dance sessions or find a supplementary aerobic exercise. (Swimming is recommended by professional dancers.) Good aerobic dance means steady routines at about 112 musical beats a minute or more. Using the principles of effective interval training, don't rest too long between numbers.

Dance recognizes no age limits. Developing balance, control, flexibility, strength, and endurance are beneficial to everyone. Some parts of the dance training spectrum fit especially well the fitness needs of chil-

Jogging and older women

Jogging isn't recommended for older women because of the increased risk of injury to aging bones and joints. Stick with brisk walking, stationary cycling, and swimming for good aerobic exercise.

dren, older folks, and individuals with physical impairments. Balance and muscle control, particularly, receive attention in dance as in no other comparable aerobic exercise.

Injuries don't happen often in dance; they're the usual assortment of pulls and strains, mostly among novices. If you decide to work at becoming a ballet dancer, you can expect foot problems. Even with the best training, dancing "on toe" isn't compatible with foot anatomy.

Jogging

A few sports develop aerobic power faster and perhaps further than jogging (namely, cross-country skiing and rowing), but no other strenuous exercise is quite so freely available. Make no mistake, though; jogging is *strenuous* exercise. Once you're past age 30, you'll need a medical checkup before beginning. And persons with health problems must have a doctor's guidance.

You can't just step into jogging as you can into, say, walking. When you're able to walk without fatigue for an hour, you're probably ready to start. And then, turning yourself into a jogger will take 4 or 5 months. During that period your 20- to 30-minute workout (every other day) should consist of short jogging intervals alternating with walking intervals, to catch your breath.

In the first week, try to jog—at an easy, natural pace—for 1 minute at a time; walk for 2 minutes, or until you feel ready, and jog for another minute. Don't try to do more than 30 minutes of this exercise.

In the second week, try increasing your jogging interval to 1½ minutes, but keep your walking, recovery interval at 2 minutes or longer. Try for 2-minute jogs in the third week, and add another minute each week. (But don't hold yourself back; you can skip ahead more quickly if these gradual steps seem too easy.) You'll find when you reach 5 or 6 minutes of nonstop running that your recovery period needs to be longer. That's fine; walk for 3 or 4 minutes instead of 2.

As you reach longer jogging intervals, at about 8 minutes, you should combine the longer interval with one or two shorter ones. An 8-minute run, for example, with two 6-minute intervals. When you can do three 8-minute intervals in one workout, move on to the next level. By the time you can do three 10-minute jogs with only a minute or so recovery between runs, you're ready to try running without recovery walks. A solid

An exercise for life

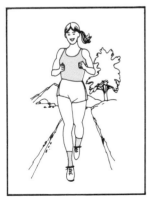

Jogging is strenuous exercise. You'll need determination and a sensible attitude when you begin. Then you'll be able to work out a program that will keep you aerobically fit for life.

How about exercise after meals?

Exercise after meals probably doesn't cause cramps; it can cause indigestion. And a stomach swollen with a heavy meal can get in the way of other organs. Best to wait 30 minutes or more after any sizable meal.

20- or 30-minute run three times a week is all you'll need for lifelong aerobic fitness.

Equipment

Properly cushioned and well-fitted running shoes are a must. Inappropriate footwear can hurt you in so many ways—from your toes all the way up to your back—that running without good foot protection is foolish. Also, wear clothing to suit the weather: as light as possible when it's warm outside; layered outfits when it's cold, so you can pull things off as your body heats up.

Surfaces

Avoid running on concrete, packed sand, and other unyielding, "dead" surfaces. Jogging is jarring. Cushioned footwear and resilient running surfaces greatly reduce punishment to your joints.

Warm-up and stretching

Because jogging is strenuous exercise, a warm-up and cool down are strongly recommended. And jogging, alas, does little for flexibility. You'll want to use a full range of flexibility exercises, but some have special importance for joggers.

Your quadriceps (the muscle in the front of your upper leg) does much of the running work. Your smaller hamstring muscles (in the back side of the leg) can be easily overpowered and pulled when opposed by the quadriceps. For this reason, hamstring-stretching exercises will actually save you some painful strains and spasms.

Running style

Always run with your natural stride length. Contact the ground with your heel, not the ball of your foot, and come forward off the toes. Your head should be erect, eyes looking ahead, not downward. With forearms held about parallel to the ground, let your arms swing easily to maintain balance.

Training levels

If you want optimum fitness from running, *don't* run more than three times each week. Injury rates soar as you add more running days to your weekly totals. For many, these injuries are offset by the satisfaction or competitive thrill of higher performance. Going ever farther and winning races is perhaps a worthy goal, but your body pays a price for your excesses.

Selecting jogging shoes

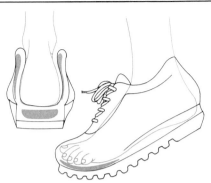

Select jogging shoes that fit properly and are well-cushioned. Use these questions to help you select your shoes:

• Have I enough toe room in the shoe? (You'll need about one-quarter or one-half inch ahead of your big toe.)

• Can I wiggle and spread my toes without their rubbing on the front of the shoe?

• Do I feel pressure on the front or sides of the shoe? (Any pressure on the front or sides can cause blisters or cramped toes.)

• Do I feel comfortable cushioning in the heels and soles? (Cushioning protects you from shock. Most good shoes have double soles—a tough outer layer to resist impact and provide traction, and one or more softer layers inside to cushion your feet and absorb shocks.)

Fartlek
When you've become a steady runner, you may find extra enjoyment in *fartlek,* a Swedish variation on the morning stroll. As you jog, speed or slow your pace to fit your mood. Sprint 100 yards, jog for a while, skip if you wish—let your imagination run the show.

Jog/walk
The training method you use to get yourself into shape for running is itself an excellent form of aerobic exercise. Any way that you wish to combine jogging and walking in your 30-minute workout is beneficial. Short jogs and occasional, shorter sprints with a few minutes of relaxed walking in between spurts make up an efficient routine. Or you needn't jog at all: brisk walking for 3 or 4 minutes followed by rest or an easier pace will also achieve good results. The combination of faster and slower walking is especially recommended for fitness beginners and for people whose health won't permit more vigorous exercise.

Marathon
No event has attracted as much attention to running as the marathon. This 26.2-mile event spawns whole books arguing the merits of various training, dietary,

biochemical, and psychological techniques. Almost everyone by now has heard of "hitting the wall" (loss of energy at about 18 or 19 miles) or knows about the importance of "carbohydrate loading" (taking on extra carbohydrate-rich food) just before a marathon. If you're attracted to the marathon, you'll have to jog for a year or two to reach the level at which marathon preparation can begin.

Tips for safe running

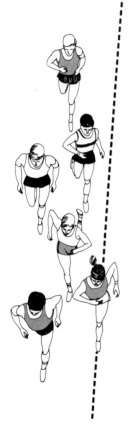

- Keep your chin parallel to the ground and look ahead four to five yards.

- Don't hunch forward; rather, keep your shoulders and back and well spread.

- To increase your speed, lengthen your stride.

- When running uphill, place your heels down first.

- Lean backward to compensate when running downhill.

- Run with the traffic.

- Wear reflective clothing when running in the dark.

- Consume liquids during long runs.

- Wear easy-to-remove layers of clothing in warm weather.

- If a threatening dog chases you, stop and confront it.

Rowing

Rowing isn't the easiest or most convenient activity to get into—you'll need access to a river or lake and a boat, or the space to use an indoor rowing machine. You'll also have to be in pretty good shape to really enjoy rowing. But if you row, you'll find it's a unique exercise. It's the equal, aerobically, to both jogging and cross-country skiing, but exercises the arms, legs, and back in rhythmic, smooth motions. Nordic skiing builds strength and endurance in as many muscle groups; rowing is superior, though, for relieving back pain. Doctors frequently recommend it.

A more specific term for handling two oars is *sculling*. That's to distinguish sculls, which are a kind of oar, from *sweeps*, the longer oars pulled two-handed, one person to each sweep. In competition, the best rowers tend to be the largest. Because you don't carry your own body's weight, as you would in skiing or running, extra muscle counts toward rowing speed. But speed isn't the measure of fitness—and racing seems somehow inappropriate to this serene, solitary activity.

Rowing injuries are uncommon, limited to strains from overdoing it. Both for the sake of your muscles and your heart, approach rowing as you would all strenuous activity: start with 1-minute work intervals and adequate recovery periods in between. Build in weekly levels, adding minutes as you progress. Once you're in shape, and if you like rowing, you can row more days each week than is usually recommended for jogging. Rowing doesn't jar or twist your body. (The same could be said of swimming or bicycling. Both are excellent for frequent exercise.)

If you're landlocked, you can buy an indoor rowing machine. A good machine duplicates rowing action and resistance quite well.

Swimming

No exercise is a more complete fitness prescription than swimming. In good measure swimming develops flexibility, strength, and aerobic capacity. For those who are overweight, swimming is especially attractive. In the water there's little penalty for carrying too much weight. You won't suffer much as you exercise to lose unwanted and unhealthy pounds. Among aerobic exercises, swimming is also the one least likely to bring on asthmatic attacks in people who're afflicted with them—but check with your doctor if you have an asthmatic condition.

Swimming is injury free aside from a few overworked shoulder muscles and occasional stretched tendons of the inner thigh (from too vigorous a frog kick in the breaststroke).

If swimming appeals to you, begin your exercise program modestly. The crawl serves best as a general-purpose stroke. You'll want to swim 30 minutes at least three times a week. You may not cover more than 100

Not enough kick?
Strangely enough, in the most efficient swimming stroke, the crawl, tests show the kick contributes little to speed. Less than 5 percent of crawl speed comes from the kick; well-trained arm strokes account for the rest. Keep kicking, though, it's good leg exercise.

Indoor pools

If you swim indoors, you'll want some special equipment. All indoor pools are chlorinated, and chlorine is very trying on skin, hair, eyes, and bathing suit. For your skin, you'll need a soap shower afterward— you may want to use one of the special soaps made to remove chlorine. Because chlorine is drying, you'll probably want to use a moisturizer after showering. For your hair, wear a swimming cap. You may also want to use a shampoo made to remove chlorine. For your eyes,

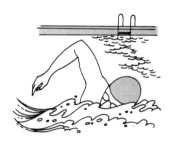

you must wear goggles. Chlorine actually dissolves the protective film over your eyes, so nonprescription eyedrops are mostly useless if you have chlorine discomfort.

Proper walking posture

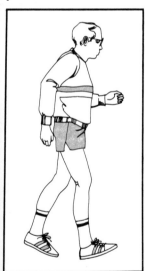

Keep your head level, with your chin parallel to the ground. Your shoulders should be back and relaxed, buttocks tucked in firmly. Swing your arms freely in opposition to your legs. A little practice is all you'll need.

yards in your first workouts; that's a prudent start if you're out of shape. Break each workout into four or more swimming distances, and tread water for a minute or two between them. The beauty of your stroke counts little toward fitness, but as your capacity grows you may wish to make a more efficient swimmer of yourself. Acquaint yourself with the best breathing techniques and smoothest style.

Please remember that even a well-conditioned swimmer encounters tougher going in open water. Don't expect to swim as easily or as far in these choppier waters.

Walking

Walking is often underestimated as a fitness activity. Test subjects, walking at about 3 miles an hour for only 30 minutes a day (5 days a week), increased their aerobic capacity by 20 percent or more in just 3 weeks. Carrying loaded 6- to 12-pound backpacks—as you might on your way to work—led to aerobic improvements as high as 35 percent in this same group. Walking also has the advantages of being available to almost everyone, in all seasons, and for virtually no cost, except the purchase price of good walking shoes.

Though walking perhaps lacks the fitness glamour of such activities as jogging, it's superior to other exercises for those just beginning a fitness routine. For one thing, you won't need any special training to walk; for

Combine exercises

No single sport, activity, or exercise can do everything for you. Even those activities that work on the widest muscle range—swimming or cross-country skiing—might become monotonous if you were to do nothing else. Combine your exercises, find new ones, don't let the fitness experience become stale for you. In this way, too, you're less likely to overuse some muscles and underuse others.

Always be willing to try new exercises and activities. And always stay active.

another, injuries more serious than a heel blister simply don't occur. Regular walking is also one of the steadiest ways to lose weight—maybe because it fits so painlessly into everyday schedules.

If you're now walking for fitness, or thinking about starting, here's some advice:

• Start slowly, 30 to 40 minutes at a time to begin with. Walk at a comfortable, brisk pace. You shouldn't feel breathless or unable to carry on a conversation while walking.

• As you progress from week to week you'll probably find you're walking comfortably at higher speeds. But don't race. You may add a backpack or ankle weights to increase your training benefit—wait until you've logged 3 or 4 weeks of exercise.

• Think about safety when you walk close to traffic. Face traffic when you walk on a road shoulder. Wear light-colored, reflective clothing at night.

• Look for excuses to walk instead of taking the car, the escalator, or the elevator. And if your walking habit grows into a hiking habit, invest in comfortable, tough footwear that supports your ankles.

7 Rating sports and activities

In this chapter, you'll find a range of sports and activities assigned approximate values, from 1 to 10, for their aerobic benefits, muscular development, and flexibility. To help complete your rating information, special injury hazards, expense, and difficulty of access receive negative numbers. These liabilities are rated from 0 to minus 5.

Explanation of the ratings

• **Aerobic benefit.** A relative measure of potential heart and circulatory improvement.

• **Muscle development.** High marks are awarded only to activities that exercise a full muscle range.

• **Flexibility.** Sports that require reaches and stretches score well.

• **Injury hazard.** A high injury hazard means both frequent and serious injuries. Medium scores, like that assigned to wrestling, indicate a rough but safe sport.

• **Access.** One point is deducted for special equipment (such as rackets, gloves, balls), and another for special facilities (courts, playing fields). An additional point is subtracted for scarcer, hard-to-schedule facilities (gyms, pools, squash courts). Seasonal limitation counts as another deduction (hockey, ice skating). Activities possible only in special terrain cost another point (riding, skiing, surfing).

• **Expense.** Deductions for expense are 1 point for costlier equipment (bicycles, golf clubs, skis); 1 point for renting facilities (golf course, tennis courts, ski-lift pass); 1 point for sports that require extensive lessons (riding, skiing, judo); 1 point for unusual travel distance (skiing, surfing, riding); and 1 point for those sports associated with higher medical expenses (downhill skiing, horseback riding, boxing).

• **Total activity rating.** Use these ranges to evaluate the scores given for each activity:

19–23	Excellent	7–12	Fair
13–18	Good	0–6	Not a fitness activity

Rating sports and activities

Activity	Aerobic benefit	Muscle development	Flexibility rating	Injury hazard
Badminton	7	6	8	0
Baseball	3	3	4	− 1: Hard baseballs and flying bats lead to injury. The most severe are prevented by wearing a batting helmet.
Basketball	9	7	6	− 2: High-speed collisions seem inevitable.
Bicycling	9	8	4	− 5: Traffic accidents are a big problem. Otherwise, injuries are from spokes and spills
Bowling	2	2	3	0
Boxing	8	10	4	− 10: Cumulative brain damage has been widely reported.
Calisthenics	5	8	10	0
Football	7	9	5	− 7: Each year, NFL players suffer injuries ranging from pulled muscles to broken bones and more serious damage — and these are the best conditioned participants in this sport.
Golf	4	4	4	0
Gymnastics	5	9	9	− 4: Women's gymnastic events are particularly hazardous — the balance beam is a chief offender. Also, gymnasts tend to overtrain.
Handball	9	7	8	0

Access	Expense	Comments	Total activity rating
− 2	0	Indoor courts are recommended. Waiting for a perfect, windless day may take most of a season.	19
− 2	0	Our national pastime is great fun, but when the pitcher is doing a good job, everyone else is just standing around	7
− 2	0	In basketball—an excellent conditioning sport— taller players always have an advantage.	18
− 2	− 1	Bicycles, unfortunately, are rusting away in garages because taking them out exposes them to traffic and to theft.	13
− 1	− 1	Bowling is, above all, a skill and a competition, and it's nearly useless as a fitness activity.	5
− 3	− 3	The position of this sport in high school and youth programs is now being reevaluated.	6
− 2	0	Unless you do this activity by yourself, you'll need a class and a location.	21
− 2	− 2	Football is a contact sport, even in its lighter, "touch" version. You must expect to get hurt, but don't play without protective gear.	10
− 4	− 2	If you don't carry your clubs around with you, subtract 2 points from golf's overall benefit rating.	6
− 3	− 2	Use of gymnastic equipment should never be attempted without expert guidance.	14
− 3	− 1	Wear goggles when you play handball, and your worst injury will be no more than a bruised palm.	20

(continued on page 70)

Rating sports and activities —Continued

Activity	Aerobic benefit	Muscle development	Flexibility rating	Injury hazard
Hockey (ice)	9	6	5	−7: High speeds, slashing sticks, and hurtling pucks take a toll. Protective gear is absolutely necessary.
Horseback riding	6	6	4	−8: Injuries in this sport tend to be serious.
Ice skating	9	7	7	−2: Rough ice and inexperience cause sprains and fractures. Not infrequently skate blades cause serious cuts.
Jogging	10	7	4	−1: Jogging alongside other kinds of traffic has caused fatalities. Joggers also suffer from foot and knee injuries.
Judo	7	7	10	−1: Bad falls cause injury, but judo's emphasis on fall technique is a great sports benefit.
Karate	7	8	8	−3: Though karate training only mimics maiming your opponent, real injuries do happen. Good instruction is vital.
Racquetball	9	7	8	−1: A racquetball is, unfortunately, about the same size as the human eye. Wear goggles.
Roller skating	8	6	7	−1: Spills, particularly on concrete sidewalks, cause fractures and head injuries. Wear a helmet for outdoor skating.
Rowing	10	10	6	0
Skiing (cross-country)	10	9	7	−2: Heavy exertion—not an activity for asthmatics and the older population. Most injuries are on downhill runs.

Access	Expense	Comments	Total activity rating
−4	−2	An exciting game but pretty much limited to players who "grew up" on the ice.	7
−3	−5	Horseback riding is highly isometric.	0
−4	0	Long-distance skating, a passion in northern European nations, isn't seen as frequently here, though it's an icy equivalent to jogging.	17
−1	0	Jogging isn't the only aerobic activity—as its press notices sometimes suggest—but it's one of the best.	19
−1	−1	Judo is really an art combining acrobatics, conditioning, wrestling, balance, and rich traditions.	21
−1	−1	Full contact karate falls just short, usually, of lethal. Protective body and face pads must be worn if you wish to practice this karate form.	18
−3	−1	Racquetball, it's said, was invented by English inmates detained in debtors' prison—it requires high, hard walls, much like a roomy cell.	19
−3	0	The development of tough outdoor skates has greatly increased skating's popularity—also its injury rate.	17
−2	−3	Not a really accessible activity for most people, but the experience, and the exercise, are worth the extra trouble.	21
−2	−1	Nordic skiing has finally reached the same level of popularity as the flashier downhill variety.	21

(continued on page 72)

Rating sports and activities continued

Activity	Aerobic benefit	Muscle development	Flexibility rating	Injury hazard
Skiing (downhill)	8	9	7	−8: Downhill is dangerous. Good training and instruction help the odds
Soccer	9	6	5	0
Softball (slow pitch)	3	3	4	0
Squash	9	7	8	0: A squashball is softer than a handball, but eye protection is still recommended.
Surfing	5	6	6	−2: Challenging large waves has unpredictable hazards, the most injurious being collision with a loose board, yours or someone else's.
Swimming	10	7	8	0
Table tennis	5	5	7	0
Tennis	8	7	6	0
Volleyball	7	6	8	−1: Finger injuries are common, often involving reinjury to the same fingers.
Walking	7	6	4	0
Weight lifting	4	10	4	−3: Back injuries happen often, as do assorted joint sprains and muscle strains.
Wrestling	5	10	9	−3: Sprains and separations, but nothing that won't heal. A safe sport.

Access	Expense	Comments	Total activity rating
−5	−5	Downhill skiers develop great leg strength, mostly through isometric resistance.	6
−2	0	Of all outdoor team sports, soccer takes first place in aerobic effect.	18
−2	0	A fun game and a great excuse to be outdoors, but only fair as exercise.	8
−3	−1	Facilities for this sport don't exist in some areas.	20
−2	−2	Wet suits now make it possible to surf colder waters.	11
−2	0	In many ways, the perfect sport. Athletes in other sports often swim to stay in shape and to fill in training gaps.	23
−1	−1	Table tennis is the great standby for rainy days and confined space. Played with skill, it can be fast and exciting.	15
−3	−2	Play singles for best training effect. Even miserable players get good exercise if they chase loose balls.	16
−2	0	A universal and international activity. With a portable net, volleyball can be played on any yielding, reasonably even surface.	18
0	0	Walking fits easily into other nonexercise activities —errands, sightseeing, getting to work, etc. Perhaps it should receive a special, positive access rating.	17
−1	−1	For heavier, regular lifting you'll need expert guidance and perhaps access to gym equipment. These extra expenses would reduce weight lifting's total activity rating to 11 or 12.	13
−1	0	Divided into weight classes, wrestling doesn't penalize participants for size.	20

Jumping rope

If you already have a pair of running shoes, or just sneakers, you can add another aerobic activity to your list of beneficial exercises: jumping job. But check your pulse often because your aerobic effort in steady rope-skipping will be even greater than in jogging. Naturally, the faster you skip, the faster your heart will beat.

Jumping rope can be either an indoor or an outdoor activity, so it's available when the weather discourages jogging, cycling, or walking. Think carefully about choosing an indoor surface, though. Your jump rope will wear spots on most indoor floor coverings. Carpets are a bad idea anyway for rope skipping—they hamper free footwork. Linoleum or wood floors are best, if you don't mind the rope marks that repeated use will cause. Try a half-sheet of plywood as a portable, protective jump-rope surface. Concrete won't do: it's hard on your joints. And you'll wear out ropes very quickly on concrete.

The choice is yours

The 33 sports and activities we've rated should give you an idea of how to evaluate many other sports. No list is ever complete, of course, as new forms of recreation are always being invented, and older sports gain or lose popularity in unpredictable ways. Who knows but that we may someday become a nation of sport rock lifters (as the Basques are) or that we may become obsessed with martial paintbrush drills (an all but extinct Chinese exercise discipline).

When you're thinking of taking up a new activity, gauge for yourself the chief benefits you may expect as far as endurance, strength, and flexibility are concerned. Add in your enthusiasm, too; that's a completely personal benefit. Subtract, as we've done here, the injury risk, inconvenience, and uncomfortable expenses.

Fads and foolishness

Sports with very low ratings can still attract wide participation; skateboarding is a good example. At the height of skateboard popularity, the national injury rate exceeded even that of motorcycling. And yet a devoted following, mostly quite young, continues to seek collisions with hard, immovable objects. Many now wear kneepads and helmets, though. A more recent fad, freestyle skiing, is compiling a frightening injury record. Fortunately, maneuvers like somersaulting off a ski slope look (and are) dangerous enough to discourage most people.

The following activities will expose you to less obvious dangers.

Trampolining

Trampolining is bad for your knees and ankles, even when you're doing everything right. You'll sprain or break things when you're doing things wrong (like landing on the trampoline's support springs). Landing on your neck can cause serious injury.

The bouncings of trampolining aren't beneficial to any organ, especially the brain. And unusual, momentarily spiking blood pressure, experienced in such activity, is risky for some people. If you're curious, about 15,000 people in this country are injured each year on trampolines.

Hanging upside-down

Aerobic exercise does increase blood pressure, but over a period of time the amount of increase lessens. Another way to increase the blood pressure in your head is to hang upside down, which does nothing toward decreasing your overall blood pressure. It may, however, cause small vessels in your head to break, which may bloodshot your eyes or seriously injure your brain.

Antigravity boots

A recent fad had people hanging upside down, using special ankle fittings (antigravity boots) to suspend themselves from crossbars installed in doorways and closets. The benefits claimed for this batlike behavior aren't clear. Though circulation to the brain is increased, blood pressure also rises dramatically. There are no advantages to raising blood pressure to the brain. To the contrary, sudden pressure increases may cause cerebral bleeding in some individuals.

Failure of a supporting crossbar or of the boots themselves has dropped a few people on their heads. Even when equipment works well, novices sometimes discover that lifting themselves off the bar requires unexpected strength, especially of the abdominal muscles. And hanging helplessly upside down is the wrong time and place to begin building up inadequate torso strength.

Passive exercise

You can't hire a machine to do your exercise for you. Electric vibrators for your waist, thighs, calves, and arms have no fitness benefit whatsoever. They don't remove any fat as far as anyone can tell. And they cost money. Rowing and cycling machines that move you fully automatically through all the right motions are equally valueless.

A recent variation on this theme employs, inappropriately, a postsurgical therapy technique—the application of small electric currents to various muscles. Although this therapy is useful to people recovering, say, from knee surgery—while they convalesce, and stay off the knee, therapists prevent muscles from losing tone by causing muscle contractions with electric current—there's no fitness value here; it's a temporary measure to help the body hold the line during a long healing process. A fuller course of this treatment is expensive and can be painful, even dangerous, in the hands of poorly trained, nonmedical practitioners. Not only are fitness benefits scarcely noticeable, but you may emerge from such "electrocise" with a conditioned dislike of certain activity—much the same way as animals are conditioned by punishment to avoid specific behaviors.

You'd be better off to avoid exercise schemes that promise fitness without exertion.

8

Special exercise programs

Exercise for everyone
Overweight, disabled people, or those advancing in age aren't barred from exercising like everyone else who exercises. They'll enjoy the benefits of weight loss, physical and mental stimulation, and in some cases, improved mobility. Just remember whether you're handicapped or not have a physical exam before you begin an exercise program.

For people with special physical problems, a regular exercise routine can be extremely important. Your body must exercise to thrive, and certainly no less so if you're overweight, disabled, or advancing in age. A thorough checkup and medical advice will be necessary for individuals with physical handicaps or impaired health (obesity counts as impaired health). But with a little ingenuity and appropriate guidelines, almost no one is excluded from a wide choice of physical activities.

We'll consider here potential exercise contributions to the health of those with weight problems, chronic back pain, diabetes, and some physical handicaps. We'll look, too, at the way exercise grows in importance as you age.

Obesity

If you're carrying a great deal more weight than you should—and obesity is usually defined as 20 percent over the average weight for your height and build—you'll have to diet. There's no way around this elementary fact. Exercise is of nearly equal importance, though. Obesity brings increased risk of diabetes, cardiovascular disease, and stroke—risks that exercise helps to reduce. Exercise may even suppress your appetite somewhat. And it's no idle speculation that exercise and good diet can prevent some forms of diabetes in much of the adult population, most particularly, of course, in the obese.

Because health risk factors are associated with obesity, a medical checkup must precede a vigorous training program, no matter what the age of the person. The same general exercise rules apply: start slowly, avoid overexertion, and work out three times a week, up to 30 minutes each session. If you're overweight, however, you'll want to avoid activities like running, in which your weight tells heavily against you, punishing your joints and bones.

Swimming is the ideal activity for treating obesity. Buoyancy largely negates body weight in the water. And if your exercise objective is burning off fat, your body can handle swimming in larger, more frequent doses than more jarring activities. Besides swimming

Have you considered yoga?

Just as appropriate today as a few thousand years ago, yoga can scarcely be rivaled in flexibility training. That's not nearly the entire intent of yoga, but you needn't practice the whole, rigorous meditative discipline in order to stretch your muscles.

Yoga is gentle and rich in technique—after all, it's been refined over more centuries than has our alphabet. And if you do wish to venture farther into yoga, recent physiological findings suggest some surprising benefits.

Test subjects practicing yoga an hour each day for 4 months had slower blood-clotting times, which may lower stroke risk. Yoga also proved more effective than physical therapy in relieving chronic airway obstruction—a problem sometimes linked to stress. Most important, yoga helps to lower blood pressure: drugs are always the most reliable treatment for high blood pressure, but weight reduction, muscle relaxation, and yoga are in solid second place. Curiously, such measures as reduced salt intake, biofeedback, meditation, and moderate exercise occupy only the third rank.

Yoga can't do everything for you, of course. For all of yoga's emphasis on breathing exercises—some of them rather spectacular—no significant physiological effect is yet measured. Perhaps these exercises serve another purpose. In addition, in heart patient recovery, moderate physical exercise seems to be more important than yoga exercise.

Relaxed position for meditating

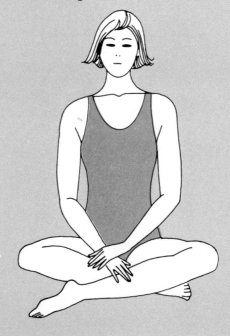

any exertion from a sitting position is a good idea—bicycling and rowing are examples. Other sports that might be considered are walking and hiking; they work well to remove extra pounds and *keep* the fat off. Sports to avoid are those that involve a lot of running and jumping.

Maintaining a trimmer weight poses an easier problem. Your choice of activities is unlimited. Regular activity *must* continue, however, as an aid to lifelong weight control. The alternative is a shorter life and a more restricted one.

Back Problems

Because so much back pain is really a muscle symptom, back problems deserve a special exercise treatment. If you've read the section about posture, you'll know that back pain and unconditioned muscles are intimately related. Also, few people are built with exact symmetry—for several reasons one hip will ride slightly higher than the other. Fit muscles have little trouble compensating for such minor imbalances. Unfit muscles, however, allow a hip tilt to become exaggerated, another source of back pain.

If you're sedentary, you'll deprive your large muscle groups of necessary exercise, leading to a loss of tone. With loss of tone, a muscle's composition changes. Frequently a trivial action, like bending to pick something up, will initiate the first painful spasms. And conditions that lead to back pain only continue to get worse when left untreated.

If you hurt your back, you should certainly see a doctor to verify that the problem is with your muscles. If it is, you may wish to try some specific back exercises. Do these once a day. Results take time, but the probability of eventual improvement is about 90 percent.

Diabetes

Diabetes, though it occurs in several forms, is a disease marked by erratic or inadequate production of insulin—needed by your body to convert and store sugar carried in your bloodstream. Diabetics learn a great deal about the body's limits and needs since they become educated about diet, metabolism, and exercise.

Exercise is highly beneficial for people with certain forms of diabetes. Insulin levels for regular exercisers actually rise, reducing the dosage needed to keep blood sugar at normal levels. Unfortunately, diabetics with Type I diabetes, in which the insulin must be injected because the pancreas is unable to produce its own insulin, cannot benefit from exercise in this way. However, since all forms of diabetes are often complicated by damage to blood vessels, exercise can make another therapeutic contribution: high cholesterol and blood sugar are implicated in blood vessel damage; exercise reduces levels of both in the blood. In short, exercise greatly improves the health outlook of diabetics. Proper diet is even more important, though, and cannot be overemphasized in controlling a diabetic condition.

Handicaps

Anyone who has lost a limb or is confined to a wheelchair doesn't have to face a life of inactivity. With mechanical aids, handicapped people can master almost any sport. Probably the least complicated activity is swimming because it allows a natural freedom of movement with a minimum of strength or limb control.

Basic fitness goals are identical for everyone. Aerobic conditioning takes priority in any training program. Besides swimming, which is available to nearly everyone, aerobic activities for those with arm disabilities may include soccer, skating, running, and bicycling; with leg disabilities, badminton, rowing, basketball, and handball. Other sports, less aerobic perhaps but no less enjoyable, may require a few adaptations—such as special saddles, outrigger skis, personalized wet suits. Such equipment, like other athletic specialties, has become more plentiful with the public's greater interest in fitness.

Age

You can delay or eliminate many common signs of advancing age with exercise. Through exercise, joints will stay flexible longer, the digestive process will work more smoothly, and insomnia will be less frequent. At any age, aerobic activity greatly enhances cardiovascular performance. For these reasons, you're never too old to begin a conditioning program with your doctor's okay. Even if you've spent six decades in relative inactivity, fitness exercise will work, and work well, to better the quality of your life. (Not everyone can start exercising at age 60 and run marathons at age 70—and not everyone would want to—but some late beginners have.)

The only physical limitations brought by increasing

Is walking always easiest?

When does walking become as strenuous as jogging? Walking at over 6 miles an hour uses the same energy as running at 3¹/₂ miles an hour. Of course, jogging is still harder on the joints than walking, even at the breakneck pace of 6 miles an hour.

age are those contained in our personal injury and disease experience. Because of advanced age, maximum heart rate will be lower, of course, so the aerobic training zone lies at a lower actual pulse—refer to the chart in Chapter 2. All the same exercise rules apply: build gradually to higher activity levels, warm up, mix your program to develop endurance, strength, and flexibility, and exercise regularly.

At all ages, an ideal workout program takes no more than 30 minutes three times a week: 5-minute warmup, brisk walks or easy jogs for 2 or 3 minutes, recovery intervals between them, and a final cool down. Nothing more is required; but as your condition improves so may your appetite for physical activity. Use some judgment when plunging into new sports. Bones do lose minerals with age—a downhill ski spill would be much harder on you than on a 20-year-old.

An eye-opening way to look at exercise for those over age 45 is to measure "physiological age" in exercisers and compare that with data for nonexercisers. Heart and lung performance, blood pressure, muscle control, flexibility, strength, even mental acuity, have all been measured, usually with the same result: for persons with similar diets and medical histories (that is, with comparable health risks), exercisers are 10 to 15 years "younger" than nonexercisers. This finally disposes of the myth that exercise somehow wears out your body. The opposite is true. Regular, moderate activity rejuvenates your body and mind.

9 Sports injuries

Blister

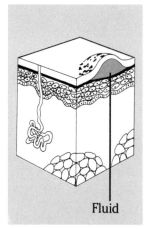

Fluid

Blisters form from friction against skin surface. Fluid collects under the skin to protect the underlying tissues. Never break a blister.

Sore muscles

Muscle pain and stiffness usually appear 8 to 10 hours after strenuous, unaccustomed exercise. The soreness is at its worst 24 to 48 hours later, and then it gradually diminishes until you've no discomfort after three or four days.

The best therapy for relieving sore muscles is to take aspirin or an aspirin substitute and get those same muscles working again. The old adage "Don't favor sore muscles" holds true. A warm bath and a massage also give temporary relief.

espite your careful exercise habits, you may injure yourself. If you've conditioned your body, avoided fatigue and overexertion, chosen not to be a boxer, slalom skier, football player, or hang glider, your injuries, happily, will be minor. Be prepared. Review these common exercise complaints and what you can do about them.

Blisters

If you know where blisters are likeliest to form, you can do a lot to prevent them. Blisters on the feet and back of the heel are the most common. Rub Vaseline on the spots where blisters may form, or try wearing extra socks, a thin pair next to the skin. You may need to change shoe designs or look for a better fit.

When you detect a blister early, cover it with a thick bandage or moleskin. You should apply an antiseptic to a popped blister, cover it with gauze, and protect the area with a ring of padding. Blister pads are available in any drugstore.

Bone bruises

When you develop a bone bruise, resign yourself to a lengthy injury. Ice can reduce the pain. Padding the area will help you carry on.

Chafing

The groin area, particularly, can become raw and irritated. A medicated powder generally solves the problem. Nylon sportswear and other synthetics are more apt to cause chafing than cotton sportswear.

Cramps

Cramps, caused by muscle spasms, happen occasionally to everyone. You're more likely, though, to have cramps if you don't warm up before exercising. Cramps brought on by overexertion or profuse sweating are a danger sign; cease activity immediately. Rest, replenish your fluids, and call it a day.

When you have a cramp, try to relax the muscle. Massage it. Keep it stretched as far as possible. Apply heat if the spasm is obstinate.

The stitch in your side

Ever wonder about those sudden, sharp pains in your side when you walk too fast or climb a few flights of stairs? Here are a couple of explanations.

Your colon, the last few feet of your intestines, bends sharply on your right side. When exercise speeds up intestinal contractions, trapped gas can build pressure at this point. The colon balloons a little, pushing on other organs. Your stitch disappears as the gas works itself down the colon. If such stitches are a problem for you, don't eat for a few hours before exercising.

The most common stitches occur around the bottom of the rib cage and have nothing to do with the colon. The diaphragm, which lifts the lower ribs for breathing, may suffer during vigorous exercise: your lungs filling and expanding above and your abdominal muscles contracting below pinch off some of the diaphragm's blood supply. The pain you feel is a muscle protest. Lightening your exertion should restore circulation quickly.

Inflamed tendons

A tendon has very limited recuperative powers. When you suffer from an inflamed tendon—actually a failure of the tendon's lubricating system—you should curtail your activities until the pain subsides. This may take a few weeks. (Most tendon injuries involve the Achilles tendon, the one behind your ankle.)

Don't take chances with a tendon injury. See a doctor if a tear is suspected or if you seem prone to tendon inflammation.

Knees

Strenuous sports can be hard on the knees. Good conditioning and good equipment prevent many knee injuries. A chronic knee problem will require medical care.

Since you can't treat a knee injury, avoid the chief causes—running on concrete and other unyielding surfaces, playing contact sports with spiked shoes, heavy lifting, and skateboards (or any other activity pretty much guaranteed to spill you onto a hard surface).

Shin splints

Many causes can produce pain low on the shins, usually called a shin splint. Whether because of hairline fracture, inflamed ligaments, or muscle strain, you'll just have to take it easy for a while.

This injury happens most frequently to runners. Hard, jarring surfaces and overtraining are usually at fault. Trainers suggest that a heel-to-toe running step is less punishing than a ball-to-toe stride.

Soreness

Sore muscles should be massaged and kept warm. Slow, easy stretches help, too.

Sprained ankle

When a misstep or uneven surface pushes the weight-bearing ankle sideways, a sprain may occur. Ice down a suspected sprain as quickly as possible. If the sprain is severe, with continued swelling and pain, see a doctor; you could have a fracture.

In activities where sprains are most likely, select footwear that supports the ankle—like lace-up boots or high-topped shoes.

Sunburn

Outdoor activity brings the risk of sunburn. And no

Medicate an itch

When chafing has led to a chronic itch, particularly on your upper thighs, you may wish to try a preparation containing miconazole. This versatile substance is often effective against a wide range of fungi and yeasts that prefer the moister, warmer parts of your body. Athlete's foot, too, often shows improvement with miconazole applications.

just in summer. Skiers are exposed to intense rays at high mountain altitudes and to high amounts of snow-reflected sunlight.

During the summer, plan to avoid the strong midday sun, between the hours of 10 and 2—that's 11 to 3 when daylight saving time is in effect. Remember that sandy beaches and water reflect sunlight, increasing your exposure.

The easiest preventive measure against sunburn is your clothing. Wear light-colored clothes (but one layer won't block all the sunlight), perhaps a wide-brimmed hat, and sunglasses in bright light. Your exposed skin can be protected with lotions and sunscreens. Use them. Zinc oxide paste or sunscreens with an SPF of 15 block completely the sun's rays—you may want to use these on areas that burn easily, such as the tip of your nose or ears.

Protection from the sun

Protect yourself from the sun by using sunscreens—creams, lotions, and makeup that screen out the sun's harmful rays. A wide variety of these products is available, and they've been rated by their SPF (Sun Protection Factor). The SPF ranges from 2 to 15 according to the degree to which the product blocks out the sun's radiation. The higher the SPF, the more effective the product is in preventing sunburn.

This chart matches skin types to recommended SPF ratings. Find your skin type in the column at left and read across to find the recommended SPF.

Skin type	Recommended SPF
Burns easily; never tans	8 or higher
Burns easily; tans minimally	6 to 7
Burns moderately; tans gradually	4 to 5
Rarely burns; always tans well	2 to 3
Rarely burns; tans easily	2

Everyone has a favorite treatment for sunburn. One of the best is aloe vera jelly; most commercial sunburn ointments contain aloe vera. Serious burns, about which you should consult your doctor, will cause you pain and discomfort for days. You'd be better off limiting your exposure in the first place.

10 Questions about exercise

As you'll see, good questions about exercise don't always have complete answers. Informed guesses by doctors and researchers will sometimes have to serve as your best guides.

Q. Is there a best exercise?
A. Just as there's no ideal body type, neither is there a best exercise. In general, your fitness increases most through some sort of aerobic activity. Whether you prefer active sports (tennis, handball, squash) or less organized exercise (running, walking, skiing), your body will thrive. If you read that cross-country skiing is at the very top of the aerobic conditioning list, that doesn't mean you should trade in your swim goggles for ski poles. Another oxygen-uptake decimal point more or less is not a fitness measure. Choose exercises with aerobic value, but choose ones you like, ones readily available.

Q. How much is too much?
A. Exercise carried to the point of injury is too much. Exercise must never become a desperate push to exhaustion. The last ounce of exertion wins races but contributes nothing to building fitness. A few moments of effort at or above your aerobic maximum isn't a bad thing; exhaustion is. If you're aiming at a healthy, overall fitness, exercise in the range of 70 to 85 percent of your aerobic capacity.

Q. How much is too little?
A. Many experts believe a 20- to 30-minute workout three times a week is the minimum effective exercise dose. Use this as a guideline. Remember, too, that a highly active life-style or occupation counts heavily toward fitness.

Q. Does attitude count?
A. Until recently, scientific ideas about the advisability of exercise during pregnancy were based on rat studies carried out in the 1950s. These studies convinced many doctors that such exercise carried risks. Yet, later findings about exercising women seemed to show no added risk in pregnancy. What happened?

A closer look at the original rat experiments disclosed a significant but overlooked factor: in the course of the experiment, two trainers had conditioned the test animals to run a treadmill. One had rewarded the rats for exercise; the other had administered small electric shocks. When it occurred to someone to separate the two trainer groups, new data emerged. Pregnant rats trained to view exercise positively —as the way to rewards—had normal pregnancies and healthy offspring. Animals trained with negative experience—exercising to avoid punishment—didn't fare as well. This experiment is by no means the last word in pregnancy and exercise, but it points dramatically to the influence of attitude on health and exercise benefits. No one, perhaps, can assign an exact measurement to the importance of your attitude toward exercise, or fitness, or anything else. Attitude does count, though. Don't exercise as a punishment for past shortcomings, physical or otherwise. Dismiss all memories of those dull physical drills generations of us endured in high school. Find activities you can enjoy, and do them.

Q. Do muscles turn to fat when unused?
A. Though the body accomplishes many miracles, it can't turn muscle into fat. If athletes do put on weight in the off-season, or in sedentary occupations, these new pounds reflect dietary habits, reduced activity level, and body type.

Q. Can fat be exercised away from specific areas?
A. "Spot" reducing doesn't work as far as researchers can tell. No amount of vibration, massage, or special pulls and stretches will burn fat from a target area. But exercise *is* the answer. Toning and strengthening specific muscles usually changes the way your body carries fat, smoothing and tightening your shape. At the same time, exercise does burn fat away, though not uniformly or in predictable spots.

Q. Can "carbohydrate loading" increase performance?
A. Carbohydrates (starches and sugar) fuel the muscles. Endurance athletes often consume large carbohydrate amounts in the 2 or 3 days before an event, usually eating only lightly before the loading period begins. This seems to increase muscle fuel stores (and sometimes backfires, causing nausea and weakness).

You should consider carbohydrate loading only if you participate in long-distance, high-endurance events. Loading doesn't enhance fitness or have training effects on endurance; it's a way of taking on extra fuel for long-haul exertion.

Q. Is sweating a kind of exercise?
A. No! Perspiration, by evaporating on the skin, carries off excess body heat. The body, like any other machine, is a long way from 100 percent efficient. Its frictional and waste heat must be vented somewhere. When breathing and direct radiation can no longer handle the heat load, sweating begins. Sweating has several costs, however: the extra work done by sweat glands uses energy, and the body loses

fluids, which carry away electrolytes (potassium and sodium). As electrolyte supplies run low, muscles may cramp. At even lower levels heat exhaustion and heat stroke are possibilities. (Fortunately, an average person can drink and lose a lot of fluid—up to 6 pints—before electrolyte replacement is needed.)

Profuse sweating actually robs you of energy. When your body is overheated, not only are your sweat glands working overtime, but your heart is putting extra effort into circulating blood close to your skin, for better cooling. It makes no sense whatever to put on warm clothing and exercise until you're dripping sweat.

Q. Will salt tablets replace lost electrolytes?
A. Avoid salt tablets. Take a little salt in water or with food if you're expecting to sweat heavily. Have a little more after exercise. If you must use salt tablets, take only 1 with 1 pint (2 cups) of water.

Salt tablets can be hard on your stomach, leading to nausea and vomiting. Also, too much salt tends to pull fluids out of the tissues—resulting in muscle cramps.

Q. Does exercise require special nutrition?
A. A well-balanced diet meets all body needs. So-called training diets sometimes provide balanced nutrition and sometimes don't. (Surveys of athletes' diets find that their eating habits often leave them deficient in some vitamins.) As you become more active, your energy require-ments rise. Special tonics and food supplements may throw out of kilter the vitamin or protein proportions in your diet. As a rule, don't use special foods—just eat more of your customary fare at mealtimes.

Q. Are large vitamin doses helpful to fitness?
A. The best that can be said for megavitamin doses is that you might not hurt yourself. Then again, you might succeed in overdosing yourself. Vitamin overdose can lead to anything from skin rashes and nausea to liver damage and ulcers. Megadosage does nothing for fitness. Claims about Vitamin E and increased energy, for example, haven't a shred of scientific support. And a real E overdose can cause muscle weakness and low blood sugar, among other things.

Q. Can drugs improve physical performance?
A. Yes, of course, some drugs (particularly hormones) have significant effects on physical performance. But all drugs incur a cost, sometimes a slumping aftereffect, occasionally real medical problems. Drugs don't boost fitness, though they may win athletic contests—which is a very different thing.

Q. Do smokers benefit from exercise?
A. Nothing can alter the conclusive findings that no one should smoke. Exercise won't help a smoker as much as quitting does, but aerobic activity will produce marked fitness

improvement and seems to lower certain health risks—high blood pressure, artery disease, stress—even for smokers. At least partially this is true because exercise tends to reduce the habit. Smokers often report they smoke less after beginning a conditioning program. This doesn't alter the fact that stroke and cancer risks remain high for smokers.

Q. Can exercise be dangerous?
A. Common sense tells you that using your body in stressful ways can be dangerous. Deaths do occur, in all age groups, during exercise. Bold statements by some doctors and researchers that a heart attack just couldn't happen while you're jogging just aren't so. In fact, the greatest risk time for exercisers is during the exercise, when physical activity is greatest.

People with a history of heart disease make up the majority of exercise deaths, young and old. In supervised cardiac rehabilitation programs the rate is about 1 death per 120,000 hours of patient exercise (120,000 hours is about 15 *years*). So, coronary patients are at risk—though a low one—in exercise. Is this really a risk? We must take into account findings that non-exercising patients die of recurring heart disease at rates as much as *eight times* higher than exercising patients. For this group we can say confidently that *not* exercising is quite dangerous.

Among the general population, exercise deaths can also happen. The most strenuous activities—jogging and cross-country skiing, for example—are riskiest. Undetected heart disease is usually the cause. (That's a very good reason for you to have a checkup before starting an exercise program.) Sometimes undetected but critical conditions such as aneurysms (weaknesses in arterial walls that rupture) are involved. In individuals with serious hidden disease, any number of stressing factors can lead to crisis. And exercise is such a factor. These deaths might well have happened anyway, even without exercise. We may say such events are exercise-related, but they are caused by disease.

Given these perspectives on exercise risk, you can more fully appreciate some approximate figures. The most strenuous exercise (we'll use jogging) carries a risk in any one year of 1 in 15,000 (1 death per year among 15,000 joggers). Jogging is therefore three times safer than riding in a car. Less strenuous activities carry risks as low as 1 in 500,000—risk levels somewhere between your chances of contracting malaria and being injured by lightning.

It's wrong, then, to think of exercise as "risky" to healthy or medically supervised individuals. Exercise is no more dangerous than hundreds of other things we do routinely each day.

Q. Does exercise increase blood clotting time and, thus, perhaps lessen the likelihood of stroke?
A. Some research indicates that exercise *decreases* blood clotting

time but also *increases* the rate at which clots are dissolved (fibrinolysis). Taken together with studies of stroke incidence, the results are unclear.

Q. Does exercise enlarge the size of major blood vessels, thereby promoting better circulation?
A. Probably not; studies disagree. It's an important question but doesn't obscure the fact that exercise *is* related, for whatever reason, to a lower incidence of coronary artery disease.

Q. Does exercise reduce cholesterol?
A. In general, yes; for many people exercise can lower blood cholesterol levels. Low-density lipoproteins (cholesterol carriers implicated in coronary heart disease) are also reduced in relation to high-density lipoproteins (much healthier kind of cholesterol carriers). But are these significant reductions? Impressive reductions seem to occur only in the most intensively active men—women have lower LDL levels to begin with. More moderate exercisers still benefit from exercise, even though LDL reduction is less. Studies don't

point to a clear answer—heredity and diet overshadow much of the exercise findings.

Q. Does exercise increase longevity?
A. No topic is more hotly debated than this one. Consider the dilemma: how can we know for sure that exercise will allow an individual to live longer than he or she would have without exercise? This dilemma will apply to any preventive action you take on your behalf. Should you live long, your having done so can't prove that one set of actions is the explanation. Be sensible, though, and bet on exercise as a key to longevity.

Q. Does exercise increase resistance to infection?
A. Though claims of increased infection resistance circulate frequently, broad studies and biochemical research don't bear them out. Intense, competitive athletics may, in fact, have an adverse relationship to infection. But exercise may be an indicator of better health—many studies find fewer sick days are taken by physically active employees.

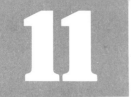

Collecting the benefits

Pinpointing the benefits

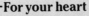

For your heart
more capillaries within the heart
greater collateral supply
greater oxygen uptake
increased size of heart muscle
more blood pumped with each heartbeat.
slower pulse, both at rest and during exertion
quicker recovery time after exertion

For your circulation
greater blood volume
lowered blood pressure
more oxygen in the blood
often, reduced fat levels in the blood

For your muscles and joints
greater muscle mass
higher strength
increased blood supply to muscles
(endurance)
more fuels (ATP, PC, etc.) stored in muscles
thicker cartilage

Other
higher stress tolerance
better thyroid function
more growth hormone
greater glucose tolerance

Health improvement pretty much stops as soon as you stop exercising. After an inactive 3 or 4 weeks, your conditioned body performs like an unconditioned one. Studies also show that intense activity at earlier periods in life (high school or college athletics, for example) has no long-term benefit once you stop exercising.

The conclusion is obvious: physical activity must become an ongoing part of your life-style. Exercise contributes to health only so long as you exercise. Since you can maintain a high fitness level with 20 to 30-minute workouts three times a week, your commitment can be very small compared to the health benefits you receive.

If you exercise regularly, you can enjoy these fitness side effects:

More energy
Aerobic conditioning greatly increases both your body's efficiency and capacity. Your daily tasks are more easily accomplished; recreational activities open up to you as vigor increases.

Improved appearance, less pain
Besides becoming slimmer and more toned, you can expect improved posture. Conditioned muscles carry the body more easily. Backaches often disappear. Many experts feel better posture allows better circulation. Certainly, chronic poor posture accounts for a good deal of nagging soreness, fatigue, and even tension.

Relaxation
People who exercise regularly can relax more readily. Perhaps the energies of tension, frustration, and anxiety are consumed through exertion. At the same time, exercise blunts to some extent your nervous system's biochemical overreaction to stress—your body handles stress more easily.

Sleeping better
Almost everyone reports more restful, regular sleep as a result of continuing exercise. Since we know that exercise can reduce stress, it's no surprise to find that exercise can relieve insomnia and disturbed sleep.

Sexual drive

People who exercise find they have greater sexual capacity. Not much real research has been done on this topic; what is available suggests that exercise enhances sexual experience for everyone, particularly as age increases.

Preventive medicine

If you exercise, you may not have fewer infections than your more inactive neighbor, but you're still administering to yourself a high-quality preventive medicine. Your body becomes less susceptible to artery disease, high blood pressure, hypoglycemia (low blood sugar), and all the ravages of stress.

You can measure preventive medicine in medical-treatment dollars saved, in better life quality, or perhaps in added years of life.

Glossary

aerobic conditioning Developing your body's ability to supply oxygen to your muscles.

anaerobic effort Short bursts of energy that exercise your muscles beyond their fuel's capacity. Anaerobic effort yields to aerobic if you continue the activity, for example, a sprint ends or slows to a run.

antagonistic muscles Muscles that work naturally against each other to hold the body upright or to extend and flex a limb.

atherosclerosis Narrowing of arteries from plaque build-up on vessel walls.

blood pressure The force exerted against artery walls by blood as it's pumped around the body.

calisthenics Stretching and strength exercises performed in place.

calorie A standard unit for heat measurement. Since body energy results in heat, calories can measure energy expenditure.

carbohydrate Sugars and starches found in foods; coverted by the body into usable and storable energy.

cholesterol A fatty substance used by the body in cell construction; high cholesterol levels in the blood are linked with *atherosclerosis.*

continuous training Nonstop aerobic exercise, optimally from 20 to 30 minutes.

coronary Referring to the heart.

diastole The resting interval between heartbeats.

ectomorph Body type distinguished by slight, angular build.

electrolytes Principally sodium, potassium, and chloride, which act in the body to conduct electric currents.

endomorph Body type distinguished by a high proportion of fat.

extensor A muscle that straightens a limb or lifts it away from the body.

flexor A muscle that bends a limb or draws it toward the body.

glucose The ready-to-use form of sugar circulated in the blood stream.

glycogen Storage form of sugar in the liver and muscles.

heart rate   The number of heart pumping strokes each minute, detectable as *pulse*.

High-density lipoprotein (HDL)   Fatty compound that carries cholesterol in the blood stream; HDL is more beneficial than *LDL*.

hypertension   High blood pressure.

hypertrophy   Enlargement of body tissue, such as muscle, from intense use.

interval training   Intense aerobic exercise in short bursts (usually 1 to 3 minutes), with recovery intervals between efforts.

isokinetic exercise   Muscle effort against constant resistance through a full range of motion. Usually requires a machine for the resistance.

isometric exercise   Muscle effort against an immovable object.

isotonic exercise   Muscle effort against variable resistance; most muscular activity—for example, body motion—is isotonic.

lactic acid   A waste by-product of most anaerobic muscle work; its buildup causes muscle fatigue.

ligament   Tough body tissue that connects bone to bone.

Low-density lipoprotein (LDL)   Fatty compound that carries *cholesterol* in the bloodstream; LDL is thought to contribute to *atherosclerosis*.

mesomorph   Body type distinguished by muscularity.

obesity   Excess body fat amounting to 20% or more weight above normal for a specific height and build.

osteoporosis   Loss of bone minerals, resulting in bones that weaken and break easily.

pulse   Pressure wave caused in the bloodstream after each heart pumping stroke; it can be easily detected in the wrist and temples.

respiration   Breathing; the exchange in the lungs of oxygen for carbon dioxide.

static effort   Muscle work against an immovable object.

submaximal exercise   Effort requiring less than the body's greatest oxygen-circulating capability.

supramaximal exercise   Exertion intense enough to require anaerobic energy supplies; such effort is above the level that can be supported by the body's maximal oxygen uptake.

systole   A heartbeat; the heart's pumping stroke.

tendon   Tough body tissue that connects muscle to bone.

Index